THE
Survival
Doctor's
COMPLETE
HANDBOOK

ALSO BY JAMES HUBBARD

Duct Tape 911: The Many Amazing Things You Can Do to Tape Yourself Together

Living Ready Pocket Manual: First Aid

The Survival Doctor's Guide to Wounds

The Survival Doctor's Guide to Burns

THE
Survival
Doctor's
COMPLETE
HANDBOOK

What to Do When Help
Is **NOT** On the Way

James Hubbard, MD, MPH

Reader's
digest

New York/Montreal

A READER'S DIGEST BOOK

Copyright © 2016 James Hubbard, MD, MPH

Illustrations by Studio Urge

Author photograph by Paul Trantow

ISBN 978-1-62145-305-5

Library of Congress Cataloging-in-Publication Control Number: 2016001005

We are committed to both the quality of our products and the service we provide to our customers. We value your comments, so please feel free to contact us.
    Reader's Digest Trade Publishing
    44 South Broadway
    White Plains, NY 10601

For more Reader's Digest products and information, visit our website:
    www.rd.com

Printed in China

10 9 8 7 6 5

NOTE TO OUR READERS

The information in this book should not be substituted for, or used to alter, medical therapy without your doctor's advice. For a specific health problem, consult your physician for guidance. If you're in a life-threatening or emergency medical situation, seek medical assistance immediately. This book is sold without warranties of any kind, express or implied, and the publisher and author disclaim any liability, loss, or damage caused by the contents of this book.

To Pam, my best friend forever, who also happens to be my wife. And to the greatest daughters a man could ever wish for, Leigh Ann and Beth. And to the newest love of my life, my grandson, Michael. Whatever good there is in me, it's because of God and my family.

CONTENTS

PREFACE

It's the worst snowstorm you can remember. The ice-covered streets are abandoned. You hear a boom in the distance, and your computer screen goes blank. Darkness. A crash and another bang from inside the house. In the hallway, your husband sits on the floor, soaked in blood. You dial 911, and all you get is a busy signal.

If someone needs immediate, advanced medical care, we usually expect a highly trained team of EMTs and paramedics to show up within minutes and take it from there. In my medical office, if I call for transport and am not hearing a siren by the time I put down the phone, I wonder what's wrong. But I'm also old enough to remember that this hasn't always been the case, especially in areas away from big cities. And it's not always the case today. If you had to wait hours for help, would you know what to do?

Almost daily we're inundated with news of terrorist attacks, riots, and natural disasters like hurricanes and earthquakes. Reports keep coming in about emergency medical services being understaffed, causing life-threatening delays in 911 response. Then there are times when you're hiking, hunting, camping, or just traveling on a lonely road with no cell-phone service and no other humans for miles. Even in the best of times, those first few minutes before an ambulance arrives are crucial. If you know a few basic medical techniques, your help could mean the sole difference between life and death.

The typical first-aid book gives you the basics. But in this book I go further—to give you medical information I believe everyone should have when expert help is not on the way.

Give this book an easily accessible, always-know-where-it-is space on your shelf. Better yet, keep it in your emergency kit. Even better, buy several copies and stow one in your car and one in your office. And read it through once or twice.

Of course, in no way am I suggesting this information should take the place of evaluation and treatment from health care professionals if available. In addition, even though this book is focused on self-help, you'll see instances throughout when I do say it's important to get care if possible. That's because there are times when help is difficult but not impossible to get—perhaps via helicopter or a long hike. If you know an injury or illness is immediately life-threatening, and you're without advanced care, machines, and medicines, this book will help you decide what to do and how quickly to do it.

This is not only life-saving knowledge, it's also life-changing. You'll feel confident and empowered, knowing that you better understand your body, some of the scariest things that can go wrong with it, and how you can help treat these conditions if disaster strikes.

1

PREPARE YOURSELF

POP QUIZ

A booming storm woke up a mother in the middle of the night. She fumbled for the light switch and discovered the electricity was out. On her way to check on her children, she tripped in the darkness and hit her face on the wall, also hurting her wrist somehow.

She told me this story as she sat on the emergency room table, drenched, holding her nose with a blood-soaked cloth and totally disgusted about the whole situation. But what if she couldn't have gotten expert help? What if the storm had knocked out the phones and felled trees onto the roads? What should she have done?

A. Put an ice pack on her forehead to stop the nosebleed.

B. Not worry about her wrist if she could move her fingers. That would mean there were no broken bones.

C. Gotten someone to find her copy of this book, stored in its usual place in her safe.

D. Run outside and bang on the neighbors' doors, screaming, "Is there a doctor in the house?!"

ANSWERS

A. Incorrect. Ice might help cut down on the blood flow, but the main thing to do is apply direct pressure to the most likely source of the bleeding. In the case of your nose, that means pinching just below the nasal bone. And keep the pressure constant for a good five minutes or more, so the blood will have time to clot. Oh, and never leave ice directly on the skin for more than a couple of minutes unless you have it wrapped in something like a cloth. Otherwise you could create your own self-made version of frostbite.

B. Incorrect. Moving your fingers, toes, or anything else might help you decide whether there's muscle, tendon, or joint damage, but it won't tell you a thing about whether a bone is broken. Nothing. Nada. It's a myth (see page 41).

C. Correct. See page 5 for more on safe rooms.

D. Incorrect. I hope you didn't choose D, unless you know your neighbors, they don't own guns, and they know you quite well and like you very much.

DON'T GET CAUGHT BY SURPRISE

Have you ever been to the grocery store before a storm? The milk, bread, and bottled water shelves are empty, and people are running around like chickens with their heads cut off, grabbing whatever is left. You can feel the panic in the air.

Others who have gotten ready ahead of time are safe at home with their feet propped up, drinking herbal tea. They've had time to smooth out important details with a level head—things like shuttering the windows and making sure everyone is accounted for. When it comes to emergencies, there's no better advice than the Boy Scout motto, "Be Prepared."

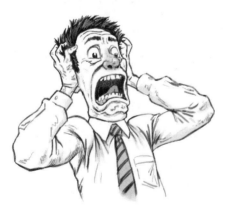

PREPARATION TIPS

Imagine a sudden catastrophe. No time for the store. Thinking is shifted to fast mode and clouded by the impending and immediate danger. If you're not prepared, chances are you're going to forget something, maybe something important.

TIP 1: TAKE "SURVIVAL OF THE FITTEST" SERIOUSLY

Maintaining optimal health and fitness is one of the best things you can do, not only for your health but also to be ready for an emergency. Aerobic and weight-bearing exercise should be a priority in your daily life. Who knows when you may need to run for shelter with a child in your arms or perform CPR on a neighbor?

Eat nutritious food and get your sleep. These are the best ways to build up your immunity. Keep your weight under control. Stop smoking. Get regular physical exams. Then, even if you get sick or hurt during a disaster, you have a better chance of surviving.

TIP 2: REMEMBER, PRACTICE MAKES PERFECT— WELL, ALMOST

Health care professionals train for potential emergencies as a team. We practice drills until we can perform them without thinking. When someone comes in unconscious or seriously injured, we don't have to stand around pondering what to do. We even have equipment placed where we can find it without looking.

Of course we can't practice every scenario, but these drills allow us to go on autopilot in the most common situations. Then we can have more time to focus on the unexpected if it happens. That's why first responders and emergency service personnel perform those disaster drills you read about in the newspaper. Time is valuable in catastrophes—and so is knowledge.

We also read up on uncommon procedures so they're at least in the back of our minds. When the time comes to perform one, we may have to refer to our sources, but we know where to look and who to call to help us out.

You should make similar preparations. Read this book from cover to cover so you know what's in it and where to look if you need quick details. Learn how to treat common emergencies. Memorize the first steps until you can do them without thinking—like a reflex. Then have this book ready for reference.

Store your medical supplies all together in an easily accessible area and check them regularly to make sure nothing is missing or out of date.

Also, consider taking hands-on first aid and CPR courses. The Red Cross or the American Heart Association probably sponsors some in your area. I offer a video-based course.

Remember, emergencies go better with organization and a leader. Someday you may have to be a leader, whether you like it or not.

TIP 3: GET A SHOT IN THE ARM

Knowledge, admittedly, goes only so far. You also have to be physically prepared. So suck it up and get those shots. Check with your health care provider for recommendations. The Centers for Disease Control and Prevention has immunization schedules at http://www.cdc.gov/vaccines. As with any medication or supplement—anything that affects your body—first read up on potential side effects, complications, and precautions.

Here are some of the vaccines you may want to consider:

- **Tetanus:** After a series of shots, usually given in childhood, get a booster about every ten years to prevent a painful and potentially deadly infection from a type of soil-borne bacteria. (If you never got tetanus shots as a kid, talk to your doctor about what you should do.)

- **Flu:** If you end up packed in a shelter full of sick and coughing people, having had your yearly flu shot could prove invaluable.

- **Pneumonia:** Pneumococcal pneumonia is a common and serious infection that is often most deadly to the youngest and oldest of us. The shot was added to the routine childhood vaccination regimen around 2001, so many adults have never been vaccinated. One dose is usually sufficient, with a second at age sixty-five.

- **Hepatitis B:** Hep B is a serious but preventable disease. It's spread through bodily fluids—for example, you can get it if an infected person's blood enters your system through a scratch on your skin. The vaccine became part of the routine childhood vaccination regimen around 1994. Those of us who didn't get it as kids need a series of three shots for immunity.

> ## Myth Alert
>
> **Myth: You can get the flu from the flu shot.**
>
> **Fact:** The virus in the shot is *dead*. You can't get an infection from a dead bug. However, some people have cold-like symptoms for two or three days and think it's the flu. It's not. The flu lasts longer and is usually much more severe.

TIP 4: GET A ROOM

Locate the safest room in the house and designate it your safe room. Keep all emergency supplies, including a medical kit, there. The choice of room will vary depending on where you live. It might be a basement or inner, windowless room. If flooding is a concern, it could be upstairs.

TIP 5: MAKE A KIT

Buy a good first aid kit or make one yourself. Be sure the container is sturdy, waterproof, and filled with the supplies listed in Chapter 14. Keep this book in your kit. Consider making additional kits for your car and office. Refresh supplies before they expire and immediately replace anything you take out.

TIP 6: BECOME A PACK RAT

After you've been on a medication for several months and it seems to be doing the job, ask your prescriber for a month's extra to keep on hand for an emergency. Some practitioners will say yes—it depends on the provider and the medication. *Warning:* insurance probably won't pay for the extra bottle. But it may be cheap if you take a generic.

If you can't get the additional bottle, at least accumulate a few extra pills by refilling the prescription a few days before it runs out every month. Check with your pharmacy about how many days' leeway your insurance will give you.

Keep the extras in your medical kit or kits, and remember to swap new pills for the stored ones every few months. That way, you'll be hanging on to the ones with the longest expiration dates. The same goes for your over-the-counter medicines, such as painkillers, antacids, skin creams, and others. (You should actually do that for anything with an expiration date—batteries, for instance.)

TIP 7: CAN IT

Have several days' to weeks' worth of nonperishable food on hand—canned, dried, whatever. Make note of expiration dates and, again, refresh the supplies before they expire. Never eat from swollen or rusty cans, since they might contain deadly botulism or other infectious agents.

TIP 8: STORE WATER, WATER EVERYWHERE

Going without food is tough, but go without water and you die pretty quickly. Make it your first-priority provision. See page 240 for information about storage, disinfection, and alternative sources.

2

SKIN—MORE THAN JUST A COVER-UP

POP QUIZ

A mother comes in to my office with a screaming child, about two years old. The mom was boiling some water, and her young daughter touched the hot pan.

Before seeking medical attention, the first and most effective thing the mother could have done is:

A. Apply a burn ointment. If that's not available, put butter on it.

B. Run cool water over the burned area.

C. Have the child hold her hand above her heart.

D. Run to get the aloe vera gel.

ANSWERS

A. Incorrect. Never use grease, ointment, or butter on a burn during the first few minutes. It just holds in the heat. After a few hours, if the burn has broken the skin and she's unable to get expert help, then the mom could cover the burn with antibiotic cream.

B. Correct. The mom should have immediately cooled off the burn with water. It helps the pain and minimizes tissue damage. Don't use ice unless it's a small burn (the size of a quarter) with unbroken skin. Ice may impede important blood flow to the damaged tissue.

C. Incorrect. While it's not the most effective treatment, having the child hold her hand above her heart might help the pain a bit by decreasing circulation to the nerves.

D. Incorrect. After about fifteen to thirty minutes of cooling with water, the mom could use aloe vera gel. If water isn't readily available, she could go with the aloe vera first.

SKIN'S ESSENTIAL FUNCTIONS

Quick—what's your body's largest organ?

The skin.

"Tell me something I didn't know," you're thinking. How about this? The skin is in charge of some of your essential bodily functions. It is multilayered, multifunctional, and dynamic. Old cells continually slough off as new cells replace them.

As a doctor, I'm amazed by the skin's restorative powers. Scrape it, and it grows back. If you get a bad cut, pull the edges close, and voilà, it mends. If something rubs or irritates it, over time the skin reacts by getting thicker to protect itself.

But there's lots, lots more. To understand why some injuries need serious attention—lest they lead to worse problems—you first must understand the many jobs for which your skin is responsible.

JOB 1: CENTRAL-AIR REGULATOR

Blood vessels in or near your skin react constantly to keep your inner core (where most of your other organs reside) nice and warm, but not too warm. If your core starts getting too hot, the vessels get larger and bring more blood close to the surface to cool off. If your core gets cold, the vessels constrict and keep the warm blood in. Extreme hot and cold temperatures can overwhelm these mechanisms so they don't work anymore (see page 232).

JOB 2: STORAGE DEVICE

The skin stores fat (too well, in my case!) for energy reserves, and it keeps your internal fluids from evaporating. Without the skin, you'd quickly dehydrate and become a heap of dried meat. A major danger from really large burns—those covering, say, 10 percent or more of your body—is the escape of huge amounts of bodily fluids, leading to severe, often deadly, dehydration.

JOB 3: SENSOR

The skin contains nerves that warn you when it's at risk of potential harm from too much heat, cold, pressure, sharp objects, or other dangers.

JOB 4: SECURITY SERVICE

The skin is a barrier and your first line of defense against germs. Like a gash in a protective wall, a large enough cut or burn breaks through this security, allowing the bad guys much easier access.

OTHER JOBS

Oil from glands in the skin keeps it waterproof; sweat glands cool you off. Melanin cells produce skin color, which helps protect you from the sun. And the skin uses the sun's ultraviolet rays to change some of your body's chemicals into vitamin D.

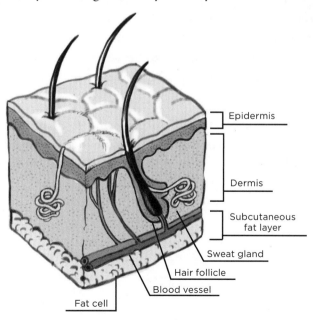

Epidermis

Dermis

Subcutaneous
fat layer

Sweat gland

Hair follicle

Blood vessel

Fat cell

SIMPLE WAYS TO PROTECT YOUR SKIN

As long as your skin is intact, you're pretty doggone safe. But get just a little scratch or nick, and one of the many microscopic menaces floating around in the air and lurking on surfaces will likely find the opening. Fortunately, your immune system provides backup protection, but scratches and blisters can become seriously infected, especially when adequate medical care, including antibiotics, is unavailable. So use the following tips to protect your skin—even during a disaster—so it can protect you:

1. Cover up: Wear long pants and long sleeves if you're going to be in the brush. Wear gloves for heavy work and well-fitting shoes or boots to avoid rubs and blisters.

2. Prevent sunburn: Apply sunscreen with an SPF of 30 or more before you go out. Reapply several times a day. Wear a hat with a wide brim.

3. Practice good hygiene: Bacteria flourish in dirt, dried oils, and sweat. Since your skin's oil is waterproof, you need a detergent, such as soap, to disperse the molecules for easy removal.

4. Moisturize: Dry skin leads to cracks. If your favorite moisturizer isn't available, any petroleum jelly–like product, which holds in the moisture your body produces, is helpful. Try applying it when you're still damp from a bath or shower.

5. Soothe rashes: Rashes cause itching and blisters, which break. Scratching the itch leads to more skin breakage and bacterial contamination. Keep open wounds clean. To control the itching, use soothing ointments, cool compresses, over-the-counter steroid creams, calamine lotion, or oral antihistamines (such as Benadryl). Topical antihistamines seem convenient because they won't make you sleepy, but be cautious! You might develop an allergic reaction to them (even if you're not allergic to oral antihistamines).

6. Care for minor scratches. Wash them with soap and water. Then protect them with a bandage, antibiotic ointment, or both. Keep in mind that some people can become allergic to the neomycin in "triple antibiotic" ointments that contain it, such as Neosporin. Bacitracin is a good alternative. Even plain petroleum jelly can help.

> **Myth Alert**
>
> **Myth: Hot water is better for hand washing.**
>
> **Fact:** Hot water does not clean your hands better than cold water. Regardless of the water temperature, focus on scrubbing both sides of your hands and under your fingernails. Use soap, and wash for a good twenty seconds. (Singing the song "Happy Birthday" twice will just about get you there.) Dry your hands well to get rid of any lingering bacteria. Hand sanitizer containing 60 percent or more alcohol is almost as good as soap and water as long as you use plenty of it.

FRICTION AND PRESSURE INJURIES

Have you ever had a sore toe or a blistered finger? It's amazing how such a little thing can give you so much discomfort. And if it gets infected and you don't have antibiotics, that little thing could become a life-threatening ordeal. Here's how to treat blisters, corns, calluses, and bunions so they stay minor issues instead of taking over your life.

BLISTERS AND CHAFING

A blister is a collection of fluid underneath your skin's top layer. Many things can cause it, such as viruses, burns, and allergic reactions. This section focuses on blisters caused by direct trauma, such as a shoe or a hammer handle rubbing against the skin.

Prevention

Dress to prevent problems: wear good-fitting shoes; wear gloves if you're going to be working with your hands; make sure your gloves, socks, and shoes are dry. Here are some troubleshooting tips:

- Customize a pair of ill-fitting shoes by cutting a small hole inside them at the area of pressure. If the shoes are too big, wear two pairs of socks. Or put a little duct tape in the shoes at the pressure area to provide a smoother surface.

- Consider applying talcum powder to the areas most prone to irritation. Putting powder on your thighs, hands, or feet does wonders by soaking up moisture and providing lubrication. An underarm antiperspirant can prevent moisture (and blisters) if applied to the soles of the feet.

- Moleskin pads, with adhesive on one side, can protect a pressure or friction point. Cut a piece larger than the irritated area. Then cut a hole in the middle, where the pressure point is, and apply the pad to your skin. Self-adhesive moleskin is available at most drugstores, but if you don't have any, duct tape is an alternative.

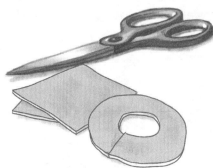

Not to worry: no moles were harmed in the making of moleskin, a soft cotton fabric frequently sold as self-adhesive pads.

Treatment

- **For small blisters:** For blisters less than, say, half an inch in diameter, keep them intact, and keep pressure off them with one of the prevention techniques listed above. An intact blister is sterile and great protection against infection. The fluid is healing also.

- **For large blisters:** If you think a blister is likely to leak, go ahead and puncture it on your own terms. Clean it often with soap and water, and keep the pressure off it so it can heal.

CORNS AND CALLUSES

A corn is just a thickening of the skin that usually results from a shoe rubbing against a toe or a toe rubbing against another toe. It's the skin's way of protecting itself from constant irritation.

Calluses are larger thickenings—the same as corns but bigger. They often occur on the palms and soles of the feet.

Corns and calluses should be left alone unless they start causing discomfort or you have poor circulation and decreased feeling in your toes (a common side effect of diabetes).

Sometimes they can make you feel like you have a pebble taped to your toe, pressing into the flesh or rubbing and causing pain or even sores. Next thing you know, the area is infected. Treat any sores with antibiotic ointment. If the area around a sore gets red, you may require oral antibiotics.

To get rid of corns and calluses, file the thick outer surface down with file or a pumice stone. Be careful not to get too aggressive and break the skin's surface, which could lead to infection.

BUNIONS

A bunion is a deformity of the joint that connects the big toe to the foot bone. It causes an angling of the joint toward the opposite foot. Only a surgeon can correct this. There's nothing to do other than make sure your toes have plenty of room in their shoes.

If the joint becomes inflamed, (red, tender, warm), consider anti-inflammatory medicine such as ibuprofen (Advil) or naproxen (Aleve) and soaking the foot in warm water.

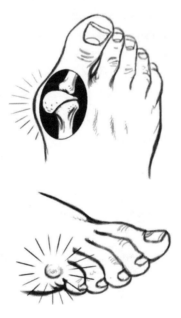

*Bunion (top)
and corn (bottom)*

PLANTAR WARTS

A wart is a noncancerous skin growth caused by a virus. If you get exposed to this virus, the way your immune system works determines whether you get a wart. It's not a question of the strength of your immune system, it's just that some immune systems see the virus as a threat and others don't.

When I was growing up, I remember that some people who had warts went to wart healers—people known to be able to get rid of a wart by rubbing it in some way. Most warts eventually go away on their own, but I've often wondered whether this rubbing might have occasionally worked. We know that some people in medical studies who are given a placebo—a nonmedicated "sugar pill"—recover from their medical conditions. Maybe those who had their warts rubbed got better because they were convinced they would. Maybe their minds stimulated their immune systems to get rid of the wart. Who knows?

A plantar wart grows on the sole of the foot. It tends to grow inward and can be confused with a callus because it forms a thick layer of skin. If you gently scrape off some of the skin with an emery board or pumice stone, you'll see a discrete lesion, about the diameter of a pinhead. There will be dark dots in the middle—dried blood from the tiny blood vessels the wart grows to help sustain itself. Avoid scraping beyond the point where you see these dots, or the blood vessels will start bleeding.

If you have a plantar wart, walking may become painful. It's like having a pebble in your shoe that never leaves. But the wart is difficult to get rid of. And if you're too aggressive, you may leave a scar that causes the same pressure problems as the wart. Sometimes plantar warts also multiply.

To try to get rid of the wart, first scrape off the skin until you see the dark spots. Then, if you have an over-the-counter wart remover, use it as directed.

An alternative is the duct-tape method:

1. Cut a piece of duct tape the size of the wart.

2. Put it over the wart, leaving it on until the tape falls off.

3. Replace as needed.

4. After six days, soak the wart for fifteen minutes in water.

5. Scrape off any dead or loose skin using an emery board or pumice stone.

Replace the duct tape and repeat the procedure as necessary for up to two months. If it's going to work, it will work within that time.

Even if a doctor freezes, burns, or cuts warts out, only about half of them go away. The others just keep coming back until the body's immune system decides it's time to get rid of them.

BLOOD UNDER A NAIL

If you bruise the flesh under your nail, there's nowhere for the blood to go except into the flesh. It can't expand outward, as other bruises can. That can cause a lot of pain, but there are easy steps you can take for relief.

Immediately elevate a mashed fingertip or toe above your heart (yelling is optional). If it starts throbbing and you notice blood accumulating under the nail, do the following:

1. Wash the digit with soap and water.

2. Straighten out a paper clip, or dull the tip of a safety pin by tapping it on a hard surface.

3. Find something to hold the paper clip or pin with—such as a pair of tweezers or a cloth—while you put the tip in a flame.

4. When it gets red-hot, place the tip lightly on the nail, over the middle of the bruise, for just a second, then quickly pull away. You're trying to burn a tiny hole. Repeat in the same place until blood comes out. At that point, you'll have a split second of worse pain followed by blissful relief.

5. After a few minutes of bleeding, place a dab of antibacterial ointment over the hole, then cover it with an adhesive bandage.

Do not do this if you don't see blood under the nail. All you'll get is a sorer finger.

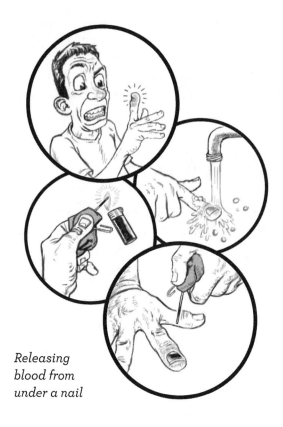

*Releasing
blood from
under a nail*

INFECTIONS

Most bacteria that make a home on the skin cause no harm to anyone. Other bacteria, such as *Streptococcus* and *Staphylococcus aureus* (strep and staph), can wreak havoc, causing infections that range from mild to deadly. Even so, they must first have an opening to get through the skin barrier. This may be a tiny crack caused by a scrape, a cut, or even dry skin. Sometimes the bacteria enter through a hair follicle.

It's much easier to prevent infections than to treat them. So stay clean with soap and water. Any soap will do. Keep dry skin moist with moisturizing cream or petroleum jelly. And diligently clean any scrape, blister, or cut and apply antibiotic ointment.

If you experience an increase in warmth or redness around a wound, or if you develop a red, swollen spot on the skin for any reason, you may have an infection. Continue to keep the wound clean and moist, and apply antibiotic ointment. Also, soak a cloth in warm water and apply to the infected area as much as possible—a minimum of twenty minutes four times a day. The heat increases the flow of blood, with its infection-fighting chemicals and white cells. Many times this in itself will resolve small areas of infection. Never use anything hot enough to burn the skin, and never use any kind of heat on people who may have decreased sensation or an inability to discern if their skin is getting too hot.

If the heat works, the infected area will improve in one of two ways: either the body will get rid of the infection, and it will just fade away, or the red area may concentrate (come to a head), and you'll feel a soft spot in the center. If you're lucky, it will open and start draining spontaneously. You may have to prick the area with a sterile, sharp object to get it to drain. Either way, continue applying heat to keep the area open and draining as long as it needs to.

If any of the following happens, the infection is getting serious, and you need oral antibiotics.

- The redness expands more than, say, half an inch around the edges

- You have a fever

- There's pus

- Red streaks are running toward your heart (meaning the infection is draining into the lymph system)

If antibiotics are not available, continue the above treatment until you can get some.

SMALL FOREIGN BODIES IN THE SKIN

When something penetrates the skin and becomes embedded, two bad things can happen: (1) the object can damage nerves, tendons, or blood vessels, and (2) if the area around the object gets infected, it's likely to stay that way until the object is taken out.

TIPS FOR REMOVAL

- **If you can see the foreign body:** Wait a few seconds before you pull it out. Think: How deep did it go? How long do you think it is? Do you think you can get it all out? Could it be plugging up a blood vessel? If it's larger than a splinter, you might want to think about leaving it alone until you can get expert help. Otherwise, make sure you can get a good grip on it. If it's friable, like rotten wood, and some breaks off in the wound, you're worse off than when you started. So you'll need to get a firm grip and pull it out on the same plane as the way it went in.

- **If you can't grip it but can see it:** You'll need sterile tweezers and maybe a sterile needle. Use the needle to pick at the skin surface to remove the object or to better see it for removal with tweezers.

- **If you can't see or feel the foreign object:** Leave it alone. Digging around for it is like trying to find a needle in a haystack. Treat the area with moist heat, as you would an infection. Often small pieces of metal just settle in and cause no harm. For most other materials, your body wants the object out as much as you do and will use its immune responses to try to bring it to the surface. If the object isn't too deep, it may just pop out in a few days. Small slivers of glass often do this. Sometimes an embedded object just can't penetrate the skin enough to pop out, so it "comes to a head" with a soft bulging in the skin. At that point a small prick in the skin with a sterile needle or blade may do the trick.

EMBEDDED FISH HOOKS

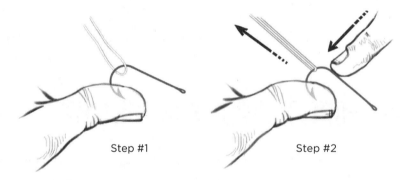

Step #1   Step #2

String method for fish hook removal

If you've ever stuck a fish hook into your flesh, you know they do a good job of digging in to stay. It happens all the time. You hook either yourself, your fishing partner, or some poor soul who just happens to be in the way of your casting. I've seen hooked fingers, hands, faces, legs, and cheeks (both front and rear).

Clean the area first. If the hook has more than one barb, put tape around the loose one so it won't become embedded during the procedure. Find some strong string, such as fishing line or dental floss. Place a length of string around the curve of the embedded hook. Press down on the back of the hook so the barb will dislodge and pull the string quick and fast. The hook may come flying out, so watch your own body parts.

If that doesn't work, you can advance the hook through the skin and cut the barb off. Ouch. Of course, this is going to damage more flesh, but it is a way to get the hook out.

If you unfortunately hook your eyeball, leave the hook alone and immediately get expert help if at all available. It's your best chance of saving some vision.

CUTS

"I feel so stupid, Doc." I hear that a lot from people who come in with cuts. Like the guy I saw who had been hosting a Super Bowl party. He was chopping celery and got so caught up watching the game that he cut the tip of his finger off.

But hey, it happens to all of us. We lose focus for a split second, or the knife slips. It's not stupidity, usually. To paraphrase a more vulgar expression: cuts happen.

Many, though, can be prevented with a little forethought. One method is to protect your skin by covering exposed areas. If you're walking in the brush, wear long pants. Wear gloves when working with your hands. When using a knife, cut away from your body, and make sure the blade is stable.

Some of the nastiest cuts I see? They're from chain saws. These machines can kick back and chew into you before you know what happened.

The fact is, even the pros who know what they're doing get cut occasionally. It's not unusual for me to see chefs, woodworkers, and other people who have been handing sharp objects all their lives come in with a cut. Pro or newbie, most cuts happen because of a lapse in focus.

STEP 1: STOP THE BLEEDING

"I can't stop this bleeding." A middle-aged man had just rushed into my clinic. He extended his bloody palm to show me. I deduced that his main problem, other than the cut, was that he had panic brain. He was in fight-or-flight mode.

It's what happens to all of us when we get excited or some unexpected danger pops up. The body routes most of its resources to the muscles, kind of leaving the brain out.

Now, that could save you when you need to fight or run from immediate danger. But it leaves your ability to think on the back burner. So I suggest memorizing a few initial steps for any common, possibly serious injuries, such as cuts, burns, and broken bones. Learn these steps so well that performing them is like a reflex.

One of the easiest first steps to remember is the one for bleeding: apply direct pressure immediately. This will usually stop the bleeding. Rather than using your open palm, wad up a clean cloth or a piece of gauze and press it onto the area. This focuses the force of the pressure onto the source of the bleeding. If you don't have any cloth, use the heel of your palm or maybe your closed fist. If the wound is on a slender limb, you may even be able to wrap your hand around the wound area and squeeze. Whatever method you choose, protect yourself from bloodborne pathogens—and the victim from germs that are on your skin—by putting on non-porous gloves first, or using a makeshift solution, such as a plastic bag.

Keep the pressure on until there's no bleeding when you take it off. That could take anywhere from a few seconds to more than fifteen minutes. Use several layers of cloth, and tape or wrap them tightly enough to keep the bleeding stopped. If you must wrap all the way around an arm or leg, you'll need to monitor the fingers or toes for warmth and a pulse to make sure they're getting enough circulation. If they're not, loosen the dressing. Otherwise it's essentially a tourniquet. More on when you actually need a tourniquet below.

If blood is spurting or pulsating out, there's probably a cut artery. Try applying deep pressure on uninjured skin a few inches up from the wound on the side closer to the heart. (The spurting tells you the blood is being pumped from the heart rather than draining back to it.)

Oozing blood is usually from a vein instead of an artery, so in that case, try applying pressure to the area away from the heart (the side closer to the foot or hand).

If an extremity is involved, elevate the cut above the heart. Take off rings if the cut involves a finger. You'll be glad you did if the finger swells.

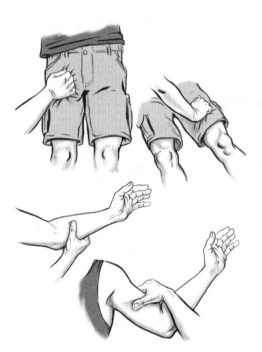

Some of the main arteries leading from the heart are positioned closer to the surface of the skin in the areas just above and below the groin and just above and below the crook of the elbow. By applying deep pressure to these areas, sometimes you can stop arterial bleeding that's beyond those areas. Practice on a willing partner: temporarily press on one of these areas and see if you can stop the pulse below it.

HOW TO USE A TOURNIQUET

Rarely, if someone is badly cut, pressure won't work. If nothing else is helping and blood is spurting rapidly out of an arm or leg, try a tourniquet.

Using a tourniquet can cause permanent damage to the part of a limb cut off from the blood supply. In fact, you could end up losing the whole limb. However, if you're running the risk of bleeding to death, it's well worth it. And recent studies have shown that the risk of permanent damage, although very real, is not nearly as great as we used to think.

Follow these steps when you deem a tourniquet necessary:

1. If you don't have a commercial tourniquet, find some sturdy, flexible material one and a half to two inches wide, such as a belt, a torn or rolled-up shirt or piece of cloth, or even duct tape.

2. Wrap it around the extremity a few inches above the wound. A cut artery may spasm and shorten a couple of inches, and you want to make sure the tourniquet is placed above the end of the artery.

3. Tighten the material until the bleeding stops.

4. To exert more pressure, tie the tourniquet ends to the middle of a sturdy rod or stick. Turn the stick as you would a faucet.

5. Keep the tourniquet tight until you can get expert help. If that's going to be more than several hours, you could loosen it a bit and try a combination of tourniquet, elevation above the heart, and direct pressure. However, the bleeding could start again, and you may not be able to stop it. If major arteries are cut and there's no way you can get expert help, the chances of saving the limb without major surgery are really slim even if you do loosen the tourniquet.

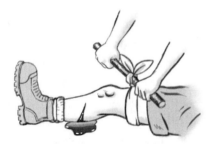 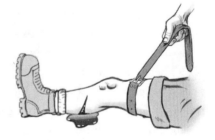

How to Close a Wound with Superglue

Superglue is great when you need to protect nicks or close small cuts. Pinch the area together and apply the glue. *Warning:* Superglue can be quite irritating to the skin. If it's ever caused you any significant redness, irritation, or itching, don't use it. If the superglue's not bothering you, don't worry about getting it off. It'll slough off on its own.

> ## The Trick to Getting Your Fingers Un-superglued
>
> Superglue is fantastic at gluing anything—sometimes too good. If you get it where you don't want it, acetone-based nail polish remover thwarts the glue's cementing power. (Don't use if you're allergic.) Try it the next time you inadvertently stick yourself together. If you're unfortunate enough to have glued your eyelids together, though, you can't use acetone-based products because they could harm your eyes. If you can't get expert help, try applying an eye patch that you've wet with water and let it stay on overnight.
>
> If nothing else, just be patient. Over time, the top layer of skin will slough off along with the glue, as the skin naturally makes new layers underneath. It's what the skin does.

STEP 2: CLEAN THE WOUND

Use clean water for superficial cuts and a cotton swab for hard-to-reach areas. Pick out any obvious foreign bodies with tweezers.

For large wounds, a pressure wash is best since soaking doesn't help much and too much scrubbing can damage tissue. If you can, place the wound under a tap, or use a squirt bottle. Water or saline solution is the best irrigant, and the more the better. (There's no scientifically proven benefit to using a saline solution, which is just clean water with a tad of salt added, but some people swear by it. And don't worry, you won't be rubbing salt in the wound; as long as you don't add too much salt, it shouldn't be painful.) You can use soap, but there's not much benefit to that if you have clean water. Strong solutions, such as undiluted peroxide or iodine, have a tendency to damage tissue a bit. But if that's all you've got, use it. Use a minimum of two ounces of liquid per half inch of laceration. The water you use doesn't have to be sterile, but it needs to be clean enough to drink.

If you have no running water and no squirt bottle, you can improvise by filling a water jug or plastic bag and piercing it near the bottom. Direct the water through this pinhole to the wound and squeeze. Or use a bulb syringe (a rubber, teardrop-shaped squirter) or even a turkey baster.

To inspect or clean a wound that you haven't been able to completely stop from bleeding, you can temporarily stop the bleeding by applying the deep pressure mentioned in Step 1.

STEP 3: GET HELP IF POSSIBLE

Sometimes expert help is available—it's just hard or even a bit dangerous to get to. And sometimes it's a lot more important to get timely help than others. The following gives you a general idea of how quickly expert help is needed in different situations and why:

- **Get help immediately** if you're losing a lot of blood—say, more than a pint (two cups)—and you can't stop it. The longer the wait, the higher the risk of bleeding to death.

- **Get help within eighteen hours** if the cut involves a broken bone. Start antibiotics immediately, if available. If a bone gets infected, it's going to be almost impossible to cure in the field.

- **Get help within three days** if you're having trouble moving joints that are distal to the wound (on the side that's away from the heart) to their full range. This could mean you have tendon damage, and not getting expert help increases the risk of permanent damage.

- **Get help within seven days** if the wound is on an extremity and your fingers or toes are numb. You could have nerve damage, which might be reparable if you get help soon enough.

Other reasons to seek medical help for a wound include:

- You're worried about scarring.

- The wound is over a joint. Moving the joint in daily activities will make the cut harder to heal.

STEP 4: CLOSE THE WOUND

If you're sure the wound is clean and you can't get expert help, you can consider closing it. This can help it heal, seal, and keep out infection. It can also have cosmetic benefits.

But there are some exceptions:

1. Don't close a wound if you're not sure it's clean. If you do close it, you're just creating a warm, cozy place for bacteria to multiply without any outside resistance. In other words, you're very likely to develop a bad, deep infection.

2. Some wounds have simply too much ground-in dirt to clean. In deep wounds, there's often no way to be sure if they're completely clean. And if you're not sure, it's better not to close.

3. Never close bites, which are full of bacteria, or puncture wounds, unless they're gaping so much that you know you can clean them well.

For any of these types of wounds, just clean them the best you can, then pack wet, sterile gauze (or the cleanest cloth you have) into the wound. Cover the wound with antibacterial ointment, and tape the packing down (or wrap around the wound with more cloth) to keep the packed material in place. Remove the gauze and repack with fresh gauze once or twice a day. Consider oral antibiotics if you have them.

> ## DIY Sterile-Gauze Substitute for Open Wounds
>
> If you have a wound that should remain open, but have no sterile gauze to pack it with, find clean rags or cloths and boil them in water for a few minutes. Cool before packing them into the wound. Or soak cloths in a mixture of nine parts clean water to one part povidone-iodine (Betadine).

How to Close a Wound without Sutures

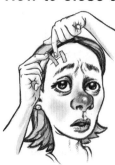

To close a wound when you can't get expert care, you don't have to have fancy equipment. You can just use plain old tape. Steri-Strips (skinny, sterile strips of tape), butterfly bandages, or regular tape will work. If tape irritates your skin, you might try a paper or latex-free version. Duct tape is great, but it can irritate your skin even more than other tapes. And don't use it if you're allergic to latex.

You can help the tape stick better by applying a little superglue to the skin first (not on the wound). Just like tape, glue can cause skin irritation in some people. Test a small area first if you're not sure.

1. Make sure the skin adjacent to the wound is dry.

2. Tear strips of tape about a half inch wide and two to three inches long.

3. Start at one end of the cut. Bring the cut edges together and tape perpendicular to the wound.

4. Continue this process along the length of the wound. Keep about a fourth of an inch to a half inch of space between the strips in case the wound needs to drain.

How to Close a Scalp Wound

If you have a head wound and aren't bald, tape isn't going to stick to your scalp. Instead, you might try supergluing the wound closed, but another alternative is to use that hair to your advantage.

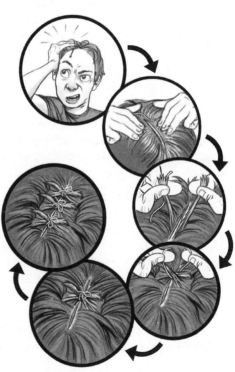

1. If you have some strong string, such as dental floss, place a strip of it in the wound.

2. Start at one end of the cut and grab several strands of hair on either side of it.

3. Twist each bunch of strands until they form two thin ropes.

4. Bring the wound together by crossing the ropes over the wound.

5. Tie the hair ropes together in a simple knot.

6. Tie the dental floss around the strands, or glue them in place.

7. Grab more strands next to the ones you've just tied down and repeat steps 3–6 (remembering to place a strand of dental floss before each tie).

8. Repeat this until the wound is closed.

Sweet Wound Care

Raw honey—honey that hasn't been pasteurized—makes a great substitute for antibacterial ointment. Not only does it kill germs, it also aids in healing. And it's time-proven. Roman soldiers were said to have used it successfully to treat their war wounds. (Note that the pasteurization process destroys many of honey's antibiotic properties.) But only lately have we begun to understand why it works so well.

Honey is acidic, and that helps kill bacteria. It also can produce low-level hydrogen peroxide. And it's concentrated in such a way that it dehydrates bacteria—just shrivels them up.

Today many wound clinics use manuka honey in treating chronic wounds, such as diabetic ulcers, that are hard to heal. Manuka honey comes from New Zealand and is famous for its antibiotic properties. The brand-name version Medihoney is also a good choice. Some types of raw honey work better than others.

You can just smear the honey on the wound. It will tend to run off, and you need a generous supply for the best effect, so if you have a gauze bandage, apply the honey directly to the gauze instead. Place the gauze on the wound, then quickly affix it with tape to seal the honey in. If the bandage remains dry and clean and the honey doesn't ooze out, you only need to change the dressing every day or two.

No honey? Try a little sugar. Just surround the wound with a bit of petroleum jelly and sprinkle the wound itself with sugar. Apply a bandage, and replace the dressing at least every twenty-four hours. Some studies have shown that sugar helps heal wounds and kill bacteria, probably, at least in part, by dehydrating the germs.

Warning: Do not use honey on children younger than two. This is because there can be a few botulism spores in some honey, and if babies eat it, the spores can turn into active bacteria in the young digestive system and produce dangerous botulism toxins. Honey has even been implicated in some deaths. It may or may not cause problems when applied to babies' skin, but I wouldn't take a chance. The only exception would be Medihoney; their product is sterilized to kill botulism spores but still maintains all of honey's antibacterial properties, so it's safe to use on children younger than two. And honey has never been shown to do harm to anyone older than two.

DEALING WITH PUNCTURE WOUNDS

In simple terms, a puncture wound is one that is deeper than it is wide. Since it's difficult to directly clean all the affected tissue in puncture wounds, they tend to get infected. So in general, don't close a puncture wound. Keeping it open allows you to continue to try to clean it regularly and lets pus and other fluids drain out, carrying bacteria with them.

If the wound area is swelling very quickly, seek medical help as soon as possible. That's because if a blood vessel is hit deep within the body, especially an artery, and you can't get enough pressure on it, you may not be able to stop the bleeding.

Also seek medical help ASAP if you think the wound has gone into a bone, the chest, or the abdominal cavity. If whatever punctures you sticks into a bone (not just hits it, but sticks into it) the bone may get infected. If the object enters the chest cavity you could have an injured lung, and if it enters the abdominal cavity you may have an injured intestinal tract. Feces could leak out and give you a life-threatening infection. More on all of these in other chapters.

If whatever made a deep puncture is still embedded, don't remove it if you think you can get help soon, because the object may be preventing some bleeding.

BURNS

Burns can be caused by heat, chemicals, or radiation, to name a few culprits. Here I'll focus on burns caused by heat.

In general, burns are not immediately life-threatening unless they have one of the following characteristics:

1. They pose a risk to your airway because your face or neck is damaged or swelling.

2. They're deep (usually a third-degree burn; see page 29) and involve 10 percent or more of the skin surface. The larger the deeply burned area is, the more urgency there is to see a doctor.

A quick and easy way to estimate what percentage of skin is burned is to compare the size of the burned area to the size of the victim's palm, which is about 1 percent of his or her total skin surface.

You can also estimate skin surface by the rule of nines. In an adult, each arm accounts for 9 percent of the total body surface, as does the head, including the neck. Each leg is 18 percent. The front part of the trunk is 18 percent. So is the back part. The last 1 percent goes for the genital area. For children, add more surface area for the head and a little less for the legs. An infant's head is about double the relative size of an adult's—about 18 percent of the total body area.

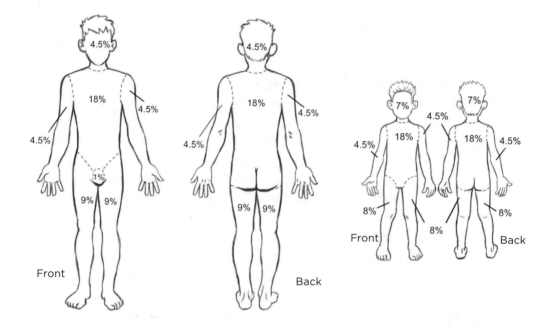

Each part of the body takes up a certain percentage of your total skin surface. These percentages are used in the rule of nines, which helps you calculate how badly someone is burned.

FIRST STEPS IN TREATMENT

The first thing to do when someone is burned is to limit the damage by cutting off all sources of heat. Remove any hot or restrictive clothing, and run cold water over the burned area. Ice is not ideal because it may constrict needed blood flow to the area.

And Grandma was wrong on this one: never use grease, butter, or ointments before cooling the burn, because they may hold the heat in.

Further treatment depends on how much skin the burn covers and the depth of skin damage (or "degree" of the burn).

Memorize This

Have a burn? Cool it with water immediately.

First-Degree Burns

The most common first-degree burns are the mild sunburns that make your skin red and painful. They can be quite miserable. I've had people come in who decided to do a little sunbathing and went to sleep with their hands behind their heads. Painful underarms cannot be fun.

Try cool compresses or aloe vera gel, along with an anti-inflammatory medicine such as ibuprofen (Advil) or naproxen (Aleve) for pain. (Never give aspirin to children. It increases their risk of Reye's syndrome, a serious disease.) Since first-degree burns damage only the top layer of skin, they should heal in a few days, usually with the resultant sloughing off of the damaged area as a new skin layer takes its place—that fun peeling stage.

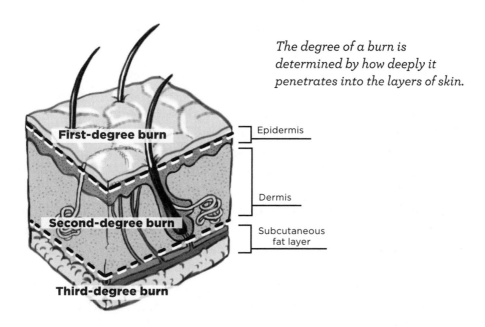

The degree of a burn is determined by how deeply it penetrates into the layers of skin.

First-degree burn

Second-degree burn

Third-degree burn

Epidermis

Dermis

Subcutaneous fat layer

Second-Degree Burns

Blistering is the second-degree burn's calling card. The blisters may form immediately or several hours after the injury. Infection is the concern. Always seek medical help when you can if the burn covers more than 5 percent of your body. For smaller areas, it's a judgment call.

These burns usually heal in two or three weeks with minimal scarring, but you need to keep them clean and protected. Leave small blisters intact, since they act as sterile bandages. Puncture blisters greater than an inch in diameter with a sterile instrument (see page 12), since they're probably going to leak anyway.

Once you puncture a blister or it starts draining on its own, clean and dress it as you would any other open wound. If the redness starts moving into healthy skin, you may need an antibiotic.

HOW TO GET TAR OFF

When you get hot tar stuck on your skin, the main thing to do is cool it off. After that, any kind of greasy substance that doesn't harm the skin can help remove it. Petroleum jelly is a good choice. Some prefer mayonnaise. Take your time, and rub the substance in well. Gently remove the tar, being careful not to take any skin with it.

Third-Degree Burns

Third-degree burns damage all the skin layers. The skin is initially blanched, speckled white, or gone. Since nerve fibers that abide in the deep layers of skin are killed, third-degree burns may not hurt as badly as others. The area may even be numb.

You need to see a doctor. If you can't get to one right away, the treatment until you can is the same as it is for second-degree burns. Keep the wound clean, and apply antibiotic ointment and a dressing—sterile if possible. Do this once or twice a day.

Wounds like this usually heal a little more quickly if you periodically pick and cut away some of the dead skin, yellow film buildup, and large scabbing. As with blisters, use sterile tweezers and scissors. And don't get too aggressive. Any skin that bleeds is still living.

While the burn is healing, it's important to keep affected joints as mobile as possible to prevent restrictive scars. Depending on the amount of surface area covered, these burns can take months to heal. Because the skin layer that regenerates new cells has been killed, the only way skin can grow back is from the sides of the wound. And it can only do this for about an inch or so. So some third-degree burns will never heal without skin grafting. Scarring is inevitable.

AFTERCARE

One of the skin's functions is to retain and store bodily fluids (see page 9). If a burn involves 10 to 20 percent of the body, you must drink a lot of liquids to avoid dehydration. A lot. Since you're losing electrolytes, it's important to include them along with water.

Pedialyte is great (for adults as well as for kids!). If you prefer sports drinks, alternate them with water or dilute them with water by half or more. An alternative is to combine half a teaspoon of salt and half a teaspoon of baking soda in a quart of water.

Whatever you choose, if 10 percent or so of your body surface is burned, drink four quarts (one gallon) of electrolyte solution a day, minimum. Add a quart for every percentage of burned surface over 10. That can add up to quite a bit, and even if you can keep it down, it may really start messing with your fluid balance and blood pressure. So being in a clinic to have them monitored and maintained can be a lifesaver. If the burn area is 20 percent or more, you're going to require special IV fluids.

Swelling can be massive. Keeping affected extremities elevated can help.

✚ HOW TO SOOTHE SKIN WITH AN ALOE VERA PLANT

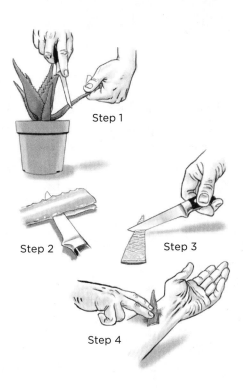

Step 1

Step 2

Step 3

Step 4

The clear gel from the aloe vera plant has soothed skin ailments for thousands of years. For quick relief, cut off a leaf near the bottom of the plant (step 1). Fillet the leaf with a sharp knife, then open it up (step 2). Cut multiple horizontal and vertical slits into the meat to loosen the gel (step 3). Rub the oozy leaf on the affected area (step 4). Do this several times a day.

Aloe vera gel is good for:

• Burns

• Rashes

• Insect bites

• Dry skin

• Hemorrhoids

POISON IVY, POISON OAK, AND POISON SUMAC

Almost any plant can cause skin irritation. Poison ivy, poison oak, and poison sumac are among the most common plants to go beyond that and cause actual allergic reactions.

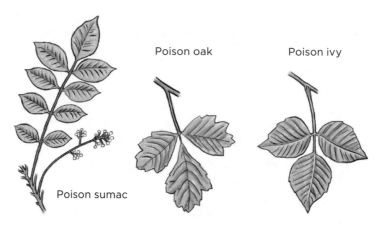

Poison oak

Poison ivy

Poison sumac

PREVENTION

To avoid the rash, avoid the plants—including stems! Know what they look like, and beware of any plant with three leaves. One problem is that these poisonous beauties are just as potent in the winter, when they're only twigs with no leaves. That's because the sap contains as much of the allergen, urushiol, as the leaves do.

Warning: If you're out in the woods and have to go to the potty, be careful what kind of natural wipes you use. Some of the worst rashes and itching I've seen have been in people who didn't follow the saying "Leaves of three, let them be."

Even if you've never had a reaction, you can potentially become allergic with any new touch.

TREATMENT

If you've come in contact with these plants, first try to stop the itchy rash before it starts. If you can wash the urushiol off within fifteen minutes, you may not have a reaction. Even getting it off four hours later can help. Soap and water or a commercial cleanser specially formulated for this purpose is best. Rubbing alcohol will do also.

Crushing up the leaves and stems of the jewelweed plant and smearing them on your skin can help also. Jewelweed likes to grow where poison ivy does, so you may be able to find some and use it pretty quickly. Just be absolutely sure you know what it looks like so you don't use the wrong plant and make the rash worse.

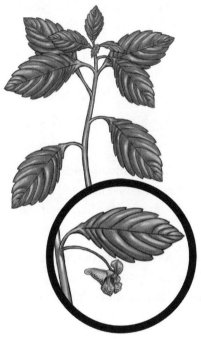

Crushed jewelweed rubbed on the skin can remove poison ivy oil. And the two plants tend to grow close by. Be careful, though. You don't want to get the two confused!

When you can, wash your clothes and anything else that may have come in contact with the plant's oil, either directly or from your contaminated skin. That may include your dog.

If the rash is coming, it'll probably kick in about twenty-four to forty-eight hours after contact, though if it's your first reaction, you may take as long as two weeks to break out. The rash can linger for two to three weeks or longer. There's no surefire cure. Starting prescription oral steroids, such as prednisone, within twenty-four hours of the reaction may abate it, but if you have to wait longer than that, the rash will probably have to run its course.

If there are blisters or breaks in the skin, keep the area clean, apply antibacterial ointment, and cover it with clean gauze. Infection is the main danger—the miserable rash will eventually fade and the fluid in the blisters will not cause further rash.

Here are some tips to relieve the itching:

- Use an over-the-counter hydrocortisone cream, and keep the area cool.

- An oral antihistamine such as diphenhydramine (Benadryl) may help.

- Try soaking a cloth in a cool solution of Domeboro (an astringent you can get from the pharmacy) mixed with water, per the labeled instructions. Apply for fifteen to thirty minutes every two hours or so. If you don't have Domeboro, you can dilute white vinegar down to about 1 percent acetic acid with water. It's not difficult, and you don't have to be exact. If the ingredients label on the bottle says that the vinegar is 5 percent acetic acid, just add five parts water to one part vinegar. Soak a cloth, and apply as needed.

- Take an oatmeal bath. Use a commercial preparation, or grind a cup or so of some oats in a blender, and add them to your bathwater.

- Wipe skin with cotton balls moistened in a witch hazel solution, available at most drugstores.

- Quercetin drops, rubbed on or taken by mouth, may help. The drops have anti-inflammatory effects and can be bought online and in some nutrition centers and natural foods stores. Read up on side effects and interactions before you use them.

- Take a shower with water as hot as you can stand (but never so hot that you risk a scalding). Stay in there until the itching stops. When you get out, you should have relief for several hours. Heat depletes your body's itch-causing histamines, at least for a while.

3

STICKS, STONES, AND BROKEN BONES

POP QUIZ

True confession time. While in college, I was working at my small hometown hospital during Christmas break. A call came that an elderly woman had fallen, and needed an ambulance. Staffing was short. I was asked to fill in. Not wanting to waste precious time, I ran toward the ambulance—and promptly slipped on a patch of ice and broke my lower leg. The woman who'd called for help? She ended up just being bruised.

Hey, on the positive side, I was already at the hospital, but what should I have done if expert help had been impossible to get?

A. As soon as I got to a safe place, lay down and kept the leg elevated until I thought it was healed. Rung a little bell if I needed help.

B. Splinted the leg and started bearing weight as tolerated the next day, maybe with a cane or crutches for a little support.

C. Sat or lay down and put the leg in constant traction (see page 52).

D. Hobbled along, trying to limp as little as possible, smiled at everyone, and hoped no one would ask how I broke it.

ANSWERS

A. Incorrect. Not walking or putting any weight on the leg risks turning a painful situation into a more serious one by increasing the potential for blood clots in the leg, or DVT (see page 139).

B. Correct. With any break or sprain, you're going to want to splint it to keep the bones from moving and, at minimum, use a cane initially. And like it or not, after a day or two I needed to start doing a little walking, lest I develop DVT (see answer A above). On the other hand, putting much weight on a break that involved the tibia—the larger of the two lower-leg bones—could cause big-time damage since the tibia bears the brunt of my body weight (see page 59). So the key here is "as tolerated." That means it may hurt a little, but don't put on so much weight that it brings tears to your eyes. Do it gradually, well–splinted and with crutches or some sort of support. And stop immediately if it feels unstable.

C. Incorrect. Unless a bone is really crooked, traction may cause more damage and pain that just leaving it alone.

D. Incorrect. I estimate that over half of people who come to my office with a broken bone explain how silly their accident was and how stupid they were. That's just hindsight. We all do things every day that could cause injury, but we get away with it. Of course, there was the older woman who was chaperoning her granddaughter's skating party and decided to take a spin around the rink. And the guy who tried washing off his driveway snow with a hose in freezing weather, then walking on the ice. But who am I to judge after my ambulance incidence? Try to be careful, but remember, even the smartest people sometimes, on hindsight, do stupid things.

ENSURE YOUR SAFETY FIRST

But lessons learned from this embarrassing tale aren't only about injury treatment. They're also about why I got hurt in the first place. This event taught me the importance of that classic advice: ensure your own safety first. In my panicked rush, I caused more commotion and wasted more time than if I'd walked slowly and carefully on that icy day—if I'd looked out for myself, just a little.

If you happen upon a medical emergency—maybe someone's injured in the woods or unconscious in a home—before you jump in to help, quickly survey the situation for dangers and take any needed precautions, even if that means delaying your aid. If whatever harmed the victim harms you, you'll just become another victim who needs assistance.

To help determine what dangers to look for, try to figure out, in general, what might have happened. For instance, could there be a mugger, a wild animal, a shooter? Are there falling rocks? If electrical lines are down, be aware that you could become electrocuted also, especially if the person is in contact with the wire or there's pooled water. If you come upon an emergency when you're driving, find a safe place to park, and watch for traffic when getting out. If you find a victim who's in water but conscious, try tossing him a rope or stick to hang onto while you pull him out. If you must go in the water, try to find a lifejacket, or anything that can help you keep afloat.

Oh, and remember: always, if possible, avoid running when it's below freezing—no matter how hard that adrenaline is pumping.

AN OUNCE OF PREVENTION

Bone, joint, and muscle injuries are some of the most common medical problems you'll see in disasters or while hiking and camping. Some injuries can be life-threatening or limb-threatening if you can't get expert help promptly. But many other strains, sprains, and even dislocated or broken bones can be treated with a minimum of supplies—that is, they can if you have the proper knowledge.

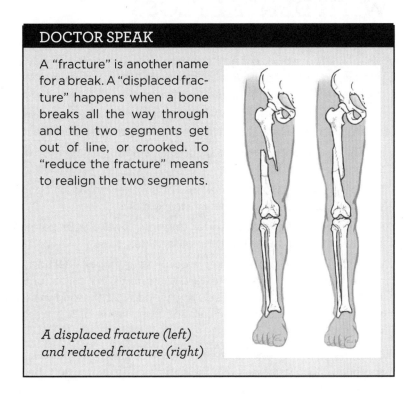

DOCTOR SPEAK

A "fracture" is another name for a break. A "displaced fracture" happens when a bone breaks all the way through and the two segments get out of line, or crooked. To "reduce the fracture" means to realign the two segments.

A displaced fracture (left) and reduced fracture (right)

EVALUATION

The most likely areas you'll see fractures and sprains are the arms, legs, hands, and feet. But unless a bone or joint is displaced, it's difficult to tell a fracture from a sprain. Both may have areas of tenderness and swelling. Many times, an X-ray has revealed that I've guessed wrong (even with my own children—sigh). But the good news is that as long as there's no bone poking through the skin and no wound near the injury (see the open fractures section on page 42), broken bone or not, the initial treatment is the same.

First, though, you need to find out whether any nerves or arteries have been injured. This helps you know how serious the injury is and how quickly you need to find professional help if at all possible. So with an arm or leg injury, always check the fingers or toes for signs of circulation and nerve damage. (Your digits are the last to receive blood flow and nerve signals, so signs of damage will likely show up there.)

 ## HOW TO REMOVE A STUCK RING WITH DENTAL FLOSS

When a ring threatens to cut off circulation to a swelling finger, you have to get that tiny tourniquet off any way you can. The quickest way is to use a ring cutter. But if you have a little time before you're in the danger zone, there is another option that sometimes works (and saves the ring).

1. If you can, ice the finger for five minutes or so to decrease some of the swelling. As usual, put a cloth between your skin and the ice.

2. Slather a lubricant such as soap, grease, or lotion all over the finger to help the ring slide.

3. Tear off a foot or two of dental floss or another strong, thick string. You could also use a thin strip of strong cloth.

4. Poke one end of the floss under the ring, toward your palm, and pull it a couple of inches out the other side.

5. Wrap the longer piece firmly around your finger, starting next to the ring and continuing toward the end of the finger until it's wrapped well past the joint you're trying to get the ring past. The goal is to compress the swelling and push some of it toward the skinnier part of your finger.

6. Grab the two-inch end of the floss that you've poked under your ring and pull on it as you push the ring past the joint, using the floss to help you move the ring.

EVALUATION PART 1: CHECK THE CIRCULATION

If there's obvious bleeding from an open wound or rapid swelling of the extremity (a clue that there's internal bleeding), treat the wound as discussed on pages 19–23: with direct pressure or perhaps a tourniquet. But an artery could still be bleeding even if there's no wound or swelling. Also, sometimes a fracture or dislocated bone has moved and is putting pressure on a major artery. Clues to this are dark or cold digits. Check the circulation by doing the following:

1. **Examine the fingers or toes on the injured side.** Compare their color and warmth to the digits on the uninjured side. If they're the same, move on to the nerve-damage check (evaluation part 2). If they aren't the same—if the digits on the injured extremity are quite a bit darker or colder than the ones on the uninjured side—an artery may have been damaged, so go to step 2.

2. **Check for a pulse.** If there is one, perhaps the arteries have just constricted because they're spasming. Arteries sometimes react this way to injury. If that's the case, the extremity is still getting blood, but less of it. Usually this will get better with a little time. If, on the other hand, you have doubts about whether there's a good pulse or if there's no pulse, you could gently reposition the injury or move the joint a bit to see if the pulse becomes evident (or stronger) and if the color and warmth improve. If the pulse is still questionable, the victim may lose a limb if he doesn't get to a medical facility.

EVALUATION PART 2: CHECK FOR NERVE DAMAGE

Using something sharp, lightly scratch each side of each of the fingers or toes on the injured extremity (without breaking the skin). If you don't have anything sharp, just lightly rub with a finger. Then do the same thing to the fingers or toes on the uninjured side. Ask the victim if it feels the same on each side. If the injured side is numb, suspect nerve damage.

A nerve injury is not a life-threatening emergency. But it needs to be surgically repaired within a few days, or the damaged part of the nerve will be lost for good.

HOW TO CHECK A PULSE

Everyone who might one day be in a position to help a sick or injured person needs to practice feeling normal pulses. When the time comes to check a pulse after an injury or when someone's blood pressure has dropped, that pulse can be pretty weak. You'll be able to find it a lot better if you've had practice.

Use two fingers. That way you'll be a little less likely to mistake the pulse in one of your fingers for the one you're trying to find. Believe me, it happens.

In the arm, the radial pulse is easiest to find. It's on the underside of your wrist on the thumb side. With the index and middle fingers of the opposite hand, find the little trough between the most outside tendon you feel and the outermost ridge of the bone in your forearm. The pulse is not too far from where your hand connects to your wrist. You'll need a little practice to know how hard to press. The ulnar pulse is also in the wrist, almost straight down from the ring finger. It's a little deeper and sometimes harder to find than the radial.

In your foot, one arterial pulse—called the posterior tibial pulse—is just behind your inner ankle. Another—the dorsalis pedis pulse—you can feel by tracing the line between the bone that connects to your big toe and the one beside it. The pulse can be felt about an inch before you reach the ankle.

You can also check a friend's pulse. Check pulses more than once, maybe in the morning and again after exercise. Get to know where they are, and recognize that they feel stronger at some times than they do at others.

Radial pulse

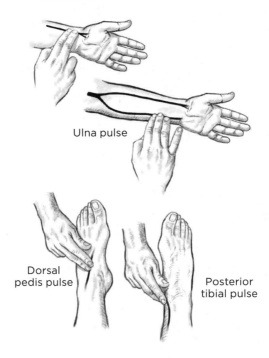

Ulna pulse

Dorsal pedis pulse

Posterior tibial pulse

Myth Alert

Myth: If the fingers move, the wrist is not broken.

Fact: So many times someone has come in to see me saying, "Doc, I know it ain't broke 'cause I can wiggle all my fingers." Wrong. Unless something else has been damaged in the injury, such as a nerve or tendon, or unless the break involves a joint, a broken bone shouldn't affect movement.

Think of the bones in your hand as fishing rods and your fingers as lures. The tendons are the fishing lines. (You can see them on the top of your hand, on the underside of your wrist, and in your foot and ankle.) Even if you break a rod—even if it's crooked—as long as the line isn't stuck or cut or tangled, the line will still move, and it'll move the lure right along with it.

TREATMENT BASICS

Whether the injury is a fracture, sprain, or strain, the initial treatment is the same. Just remember the mnemonic RICES:

- **Rest:** Using a body part that's injured can make the injury worse. If the injury is to an arm, consider putting it in a sling. If a leg or foot is hurt, stay off it as much as possible for at least a day or two, and use a cane or crutches while you're walking. Remaining immobile for long may put you at risk of DVT (see page 139), so you do want to do some walking. But if putting weight on the injury causes severe pain or it feels like the bone is moving, stop.

- **Ice:** For swelling and pain relief, apply ice for about fifteen minutes at frequent intervals. To avoid freezing the skin, put the ice and a little water in a plastic bag and place a cloth between the bag and the injured area.

- **Compression:** Wrap the injury with an elastic bandage to limit swelling. Make sure the bandage is not so tight that it cuts off circulation.

- **Elevation:** Position the injured area level with or above your heart to decrease swelling and pain.

- **Stabilization:** If you suspect a break or a bad sprain you'll need a splint to keep the injured bone or joint from moving. If a bone or joint is obviously displaced to the point where you suspect circulation or nerve damage, and if medical help is more than a few hours away, first try to put the injured area in a more natural position to take the pressure off, and then splint it.

What's the Problem with Swelling?

Swelling is your body's effort to treat an injury by stabilizing it. Swelling becomes a problem, however, when it presses on the nerves and becomes painful— or when it gets to the point of cutting off blood circulation and damaging nerves.

SPLINTING BASICS

I've seen people come in to my clinic with arms and legs wrapped in towels or splinted with cardboard, plastic, metal, or a slab of wood. Any of these can work. But the ideal splint is one that has a mixture of firmness and conformability.

You can achieve this mixture by putting soft, conformable padding, such as a blanket, a pillow, or foam, between the stiff material you're using to stabilize the injury and the body part. Make sure the padding is smooth and there are no areas of rubbing or pressure, which may injure the skin or the soft tissue beneath it.

When placing the splint, if a joint is involved in the injury, include at least one uninjured bone on each side of the injury. For example, for an injured knee, include part of the thigh and part of the lower leg in the splint. This helps stabilize the hurt area. Place the splint so you can still see the end of the extremity—at least the hand or foot. This allows you to periodically check for adequate circulation.

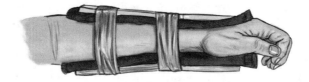

SPECIAL CONSIDERATION: OPEN FRACTURE

You're dealing with an open fracture if the broken bone has pierced through the skin. This type of injury, which can be quite disconcerting, is always serious because of the high risk of bone infection, so seek expert medical care as soon as that becomes possible.

Even if you don't see bone, suspect an open fracture if there are any flesh wounds close to the break. The bone may have pierced the skin before returning inside.

If the bone is exposed, keep it moist and covered, and splint it as is. If help is not imminent, clean the bone thoroughly. The best way to do this is to pick out any debris, then squirt the wound with clean water again and again. Use, say, twenty ounces of water for each inch of open wound.

Then you have a dilemma. If you put the bone back in place (see the traction box on page 52) it's going to be even more prone to infection, but at some point, if help is not coming, you may have to chance it, because otherwise it can't heal.

COMMON FRACTURES AND OTHER BONE INJURIES AND HOW TO TREAT THEM

The goals for treating closed fractures (meaning the bone hasn't pierced the skin) are to limit nerve damage, maintain circulation, and preserve function as much as possible. So splint it and wrap it, or even wrap it to another body part—anything you can do to keep it from moving and therefore prevent additional damage.

RIB FRACTURE

When someone tells me he's been a bull rider, I know the list of his past broken bones is going to fill an entire page. Many, though, have told me that breaking ribs was the most painful of all the injuries they sustained.

Suspect a rib fracture if there's been a direct blow to the chest and pressing on a rib hurts. Press each rib gently. If there's no pain, you could try pressing a little harder, but be careful not to push too hard. A give or crunch certainly tells you a rib is broken, but you don't want to use full force and push it out of place.

Without an X-ray, that's the best you're going to be able to do in terms of diagnosis. Fortunately, whether a bone is fractured or the chest wall is just bruised, the basic treatment's the same. Then why bother to check? If you suspect a fracture, the victim should be a little more careful with activities so the fracture doesn't move. Also, you can predict the pain will likely last four to six weeks, at a minimum. With only a bruise, the pain is usually a lot better within a couple of weeks.

In either case, you're going to want to listen to the lungs (see page 150), because there could be some internal bleeding or a collapsed lung. If a rib is broken, a piece of the bone could directly puncture a blood vessel or lung.

Treatment

Just a few years ago, doctors treated broken ribs by wrapping the rib cage, but that's now thought to potentially cause more problems—by inhibiting deep breaths—than it helps. So these days, the only thing you can do is try to diminish the pain and limit complications, such as pneumonia.

Pain medicine, ice, heat, and limiting vigorous activity may help. And make sure the injured person is taking deep breaths. In fact, she should purposely take a few every few minutes. Shallow breathing increases your risk of pneumonia. Suppressing a cough also puts you at risk. Before a cough or sneeze, have the victim hold the area that hurts with her hands or push up against a wall. Trust me: she'll be glad she did.

Flail Chest

A flail chest is a condition that occurs when several adjacent ribs are broken on the same side of the chest and each rib is broken in two or more places. This makes a square or rectangle of ribs that isn't connected to the chest wall.

When your chest expands while breathing, this area does not. This severely impairs the lung on that side and is a true emergency. Expert medical care can be lifesaving. Placing a hand or taping some padding lightly over the area of injury may help a bit. Don't tape it down tight, however, or you may impair breathing even more than doing nothing would.

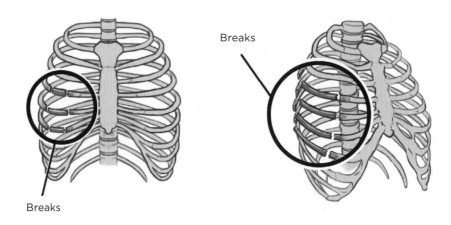

Flail chest. Notice each injured rib is broken in two places.

CLAVICLE (COLLARBONE) FRACTURE

A clavicle fracture usually results from a direct hit to the clavicle or a fall on an outstretched arm. It's a common football injury. It also often happens when someone falls and the shoulder directly hits a hard object, such as a tree.

A clavicle fracture can cause major nerve or artery damage; sometimes, the broken bone punctures the lung or skin. These are all quite rare, but if one of them does happen, try your best to get immediate expert care.

But for the typical fracture, a figure-of-eight splint or a sling is usually all that's needed immediately. Most clavicle fractures heal on their own within four to six weeks. Others may need surgery to heal properly.

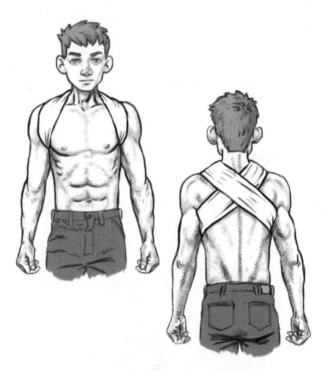

Devise a figure-of-eight brace out of any strong material, such as cloth or a wide strap or seatbelt. Tighten and tie or pin it anywhere on the loop. The goal is to pull the shoulders back and keep them that way to stabilize the broken bone.

Use a Sling for Comfort and Convenience

A sling provides comfort and elevation. You can use one for a cut, bruise, broken bone, or sprain. A sling can also be part of treatment for a shoulder joint, upper arm, or clavicle fracture, as well as an AC separation. In these cases, the sling keeps the injury still so it can heal.

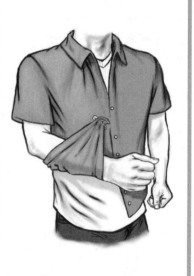

Any strong, flexible material makes a good sling. An easy way to create one is to wrap your shirttail up around your arm and fasten it to the upper part of your shirt with safety pins.

ACROMIOCLAVICULAR (AC) JOINT SPRAIN OR SEPARATION

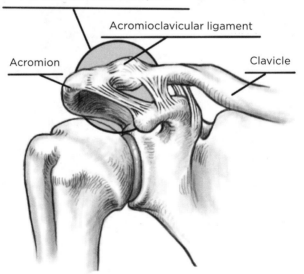

Acromioclavicular (AC) joint

Acromioclavicular ligament

Acromion

Clavicle

AC joint

Feel along your clavicle, starting close to your neck. As you get close to the shoulder you'll come upon a little knot. That's your AC joint—where your clavicle and a part of your shoulder bone called the acromion come together. As in other joints, ligaments attach these bones together, but this joint, unlike most others, doesn't move.

The usual cause of injury to an AC joint is a direct blow that stretches or tears the ligaments. By definition, that's a sprain. Swelling can separate the bones a fraction of an inch; that's called an AC separation. A full ligament tear causes full bone displacement.

Until you can get to a doctor, the treatment for any of these problems is a sling and maybe ice for the swelling. As soon as the discomfort wanes, you can start using the joint as much as you can tolerate. The area should heal in about one to six weeks, depending on the severity of the injury. If you can get expert medical help, treatment will be customized to the injury. A full tear may need surgery.

HUMERUS (UPPER ARM) FRACTURE

As a general rule, unless you have really big muscles, the entire humerus bone is pretty easy to feel. If there's a definite tender spot on the bone after an injury, suspect a fracture. The treatment, until you can get expert help, is a sling and swath, which is a sling plus a horizontal wrap to hold the arm close to the body. Even if the bone is displaced, the pull of gravity usually straightens it out over time.

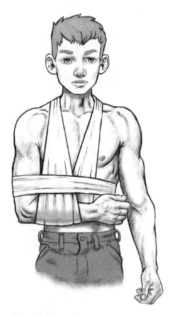

Sling and swath

SHOULDER DISLOCATION

You're slipping down a hill and grab a tree limb to stop yourself. A nice way to break a fall. But a good way to dislocate your shoulder.

Shoulder dislocations usually occur when you grab something over your head while your full body weight is being pulled downward, or when you break a forward fall with your outstretched arm. Since the shoulder is a ball-and-socket joint, if the ball gets jerked out of the socket and doesn't go straight back in, muscles and ligaments pull it back tight against the side of the lip of the socket. And there it's stuck.

For the treatment, well, think about trying to put a ball into a cup. If the ball is stuck tight to the outside part of the cup, there's no way to get it back in without unsticking the ball or breaking the cup. And if you have a dislocated shoulder, you sure don't want to break the cup.

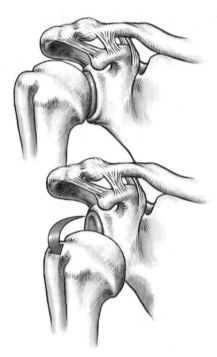

Normal shoulder (top) and dislocated shoulder (bottom)

Diagnosis

Sometimes a dislocation isn't visually obvious, even when you compare the injured side to the noninjured side. But if someone's shoulder is hurting and is hard to move, the cause of the injury can give you a clue about whether it's dislocated.

If you're unsure, have the victim touch the opposite shoulder with the fingers on his injured side. Someone with a shoulder dislocation won't be able to do this. Of course, someone with a break or just a bruise may not be able to do this, either, but if the victim *can* do it, there's no dislocation.

Treatment: Do No Harm

The best way to try to get the joint back in place is to find a way for those shoulder muscles and ligaments to relax just enough so the head of the humerus can slip over the rim of the shoulder cup and back into position. Yeah—easier said than done.

Injured muscles tend to spasm. With time they swell and stiffen even more. So in general, the quicker the joint is put back into place the easier it is to do. However, without an X-ray, dislocation or not, you really can't tell if a bone is broken or, if so, how badly. So remember the first axiom of treatment: "Do no harm." Never force anything.

Until you can get expert care, place the arm in a sling for comfort and apply ice packs or just hold the arm. If help is not going to be available soon, you could try one of the following three treatment options. Even if they work, you should keep the arm in a sling for several weeks, gradually moving and getting range of motion back while giving the muscles and ligaments time to heal.

Treatment Option 1: Arm Hang

This is the simplest method, with the least chance of additional injury.

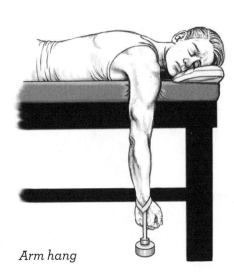

Arm hang

1. Have the injured person lie facedown on a table, bed, or something else high enough for the arm to hang off the side without touching the floor. The entire arm should hang straight down from the injured shoulder.

2. Tape or wrap a weight, ideally approximately fifteen pounds, to the hand or lower arm. (A gallon of water is about eight pounds.) Having the victim hold the weight in his hand doesn't work nearly as well, because to grip an object, you have to tense some muscles.

Soon, the victim should start to relax a bit, realizing that this procedure is not causing any additional pain. As the muscles relax, the head of the humerus will drop below the rim of the socket enough to snap back into place. Usually, the victim will hear or feel a soft pop or just experience a sudden relief of pain, but sometimes it's too gradual to sense.

If you're uncertain about whether the treatment has worked, take the weight off after about twenty minutes and see if the victim can touch his fingers to the opposite shoulder. If he can, the joint is back in place.

Treatment Option 2: Arm Pull

1. Have the victim lie on his back on a firm surface.

2. Slowly guide the arm on the injured side horizontally away from the body until it's about forty-five degrees from his side. Never force.

3. Grab the hand and pull it toward you firmly and steadily, staying in that forty-five-degree angle. You're trying to get the muscle to give just enough that the head of the humerus moves beyond the lip of the shoulder cup. If you need a little leverage, use your foot to push against the victim's side, as shown in the illustration.

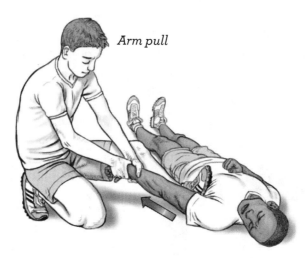

Arm pull

Treatment Option 3: Arm Rotation

This method produces some strong torque—enough to actually break a bone. So never jerk. Never force. And only use this option if expert help will be unavailable for days.

1. While the victim is lying on his back on a firm surface with his injured arm close to his body, slowly and gently rotate the forearm until the hand is faceup.

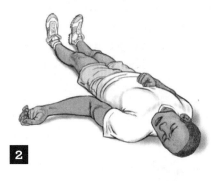

2. While keeping the humerus (upper arm) fairly close to the side of the body, bend the arm at the elbow and rotate the forearm to the side until it's at a ninety-degree angle relative to the upper arm. It should still be on the ground or table (or close to it).

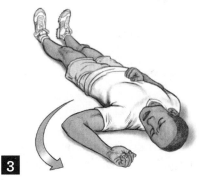

3. Keeping the elbow at this angle, move the humerus away from the body and toward the head until the hand is a little above the height of the head and the humerus is at a ninety-degree angle relative to the chest. It will look as if the victim is about to pitch a baseball.

4. Continuing to keep the elbow flexed and locked, move the forearm above the head, resting it on top of the head.

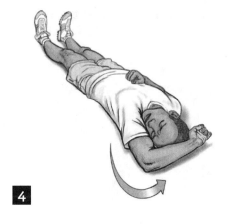

If this doesn't work, you've given it your best shot, so just reposition the arm however it's most comfortable. Place it in a sling, too, if that helps. Maybe try again after some pain medicine or a little alcohol (for the victim), but not both.

Some claim that if a person with a dislocated shoulder can just relax enough (a lot) and let the arm hang down while he's standing, the muscles will loosen enough for the shoulder to go back into place on its own. It's worth a try, but I find most people can't relax that much when they're in pain. Maybe you can.

One method I would never try is going all Rambo and banging your shoulder against a wall or tree. Yeah, I've heard some people claim it works. But you're likely to do more harm than good.

STICKS, STONES, AND BROKEN BONES

ELBOW FRACTURE

Have you ever hit your funny bone and felt that tingling all the way down into your little finger? It's really not so funny. And the "bone" isn't even a bone. It's the ulnar nerve. You can actually feel the nerve in the crevice on the inside of your elbow.

It's one of many things that pass through the elbow. In order to get to the forearms, hands, and fingers, all things—including nerves and blood vessels—must go by this little joint. So when the elbow is badly injured, too much elbow swelling could severely damage the strength and feeling downstream.

HOW TO APPLY TRACTION

Applying traction to a broken or dislocated bone involves using a pulling technique to try to straighten it.

1. Get a firm grip on the hand or foot or tips of the fingers or toes— somewhere beyond the injured part.

2. Start the pull gently, then gradually increase the force you're exerting. Always pull in the same plane as the normal anatomy of the bone. Never jerk or force. The goal is to stretch the muscles enough for the bone to be able to move back into position. In breaks, the alignment will seldom be perfect, just better.

3. After traction, the area must be splinted to keep the bone in place.

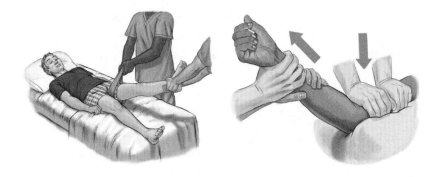

If you cannot feel a radial pulse (located in the wrist), try slightly bending and straightening the elbow until you do. If a pulse can be felt after repositioning, splint the joint in that position and place the arm in a sling.

If the repositioning doesn't work, apply traction as depicted in the middle illustration on page 54. You've done your job if you can feel a pulse. If there's no way to hang the arm off the table, like in the illustration, position the elbow to 90 degrees and pull in the same direction as shown in the drawing. If you still can't feel a pulse, reposition a little and try again. If there's no still no pulse, immediate emergency care is needed if at all possible.

In addition to checking the circulation, check for nerve damage by asking the victim if she has numbness in any part of her fingers or hands. If she does, expert care is needed soon. Also do these tests to check for nerve damage:

1. Make sure the victim can flex her thumb toward her palm and can do the thumbs-up sign.

2. See if she can bring her thumb and index finger together, forming an O.

3. Have her wrap the all her fingers around her thumb. Make sure the thumb is moving properly, not just the other fingers.

4. See if she can extend all her fingers and spread them apart.

Pain while doing these movements is not a sign of nerve damage, but inability to do them because of muscle weakness is.

Swelling can also compress a nerve or blood vessel, so with any elbow injury, consider applying an ice pack (with a cloth placed between skin and the pack) for about ten minutes on and ten minutes off. Elevate the elbow to heart level.

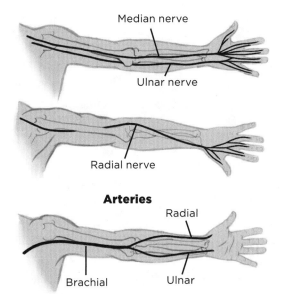

Nerves

Median nerve

Ulnar nerve

Radial nerve

Arteries

Radial

Brachial

Ulnar

The major nerves and arteries of the arm

ELBOW DISLOCATION

Although an elbow dislocation is less common than a shoulder dislocation, it's pretty obvious what's happened from just looking at the elbow. If there's any question, compare it to the uninjured side. Elbow dislocation most frequently occurs when someone falls on an outstretched arm.

Check the radial pulse in the wrist. If there is none, the limb is in danger and immediate help is essential if at all possible.

Figuring out whether there's a break in the bone in addition to the dislocation can be a little tricky, because the whole area will be tender. A clue can be a crunching sound or sensation when you apply light pressure to one of the elbow bones.

If you don't suspect a break and no medical care is available, you can try putting the joint back in place by doing the following. These steps may also help get a pulse back if there isn't one.

1. Have the victim lie facedown on a bed or table. The upper arm should be on the table and the elbow bent so that the forearm hangs free and as straight down as possible.

2. Grip the forearm. Apply gentle downward pressure for about five to ten minutes.

3. Regardless of whether your relocation effort was successful, place a ninety-degree-angled splint over the back of the upper and lower arm. Wrap the splinted arm and place it in a sling.

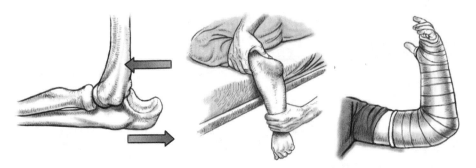

Elbow dislocation

WRIST OR HAND FRACTURE

Even if a broken hand or wrist bone is displaced, splint it as is until you can get expert care. If that's not an option and the displacement is more than a little noticeable, you can try traction (see page 52). Traction often doesn't work as well on hand fractures, though, so you may just have to live with a permanent displacement.

FINGER OR TOE FRACTURE

Splint a broken finger or toe by taping it to an adjacent uninjured digit with a little cotton padding in between. This is called a buddy splint. If the broken bone is really crooked, try traction for a few minutes first.

For a broken finger, an alternative to the buddy splint is to hold a wad of some sort of cloth—or even a soda can—with the injured hand. Curl all your fingers around it in a light grip. Wrap the whole hand with more cloth and tape or tie it so it stays on. This is a good technique if more than one finger is broken.

DISLOCATED FINGER

To treat a dislocated finger, grab the tip and apply traction. At the same time, gently push on the dislocated bone with your thumb in the same outward direction as the pulling. After the joint is back in place, tape the fingers together with a buddy splint (see above).

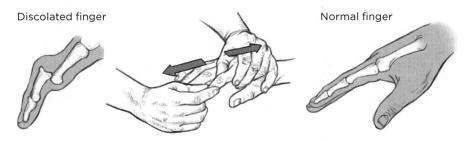

Applying traction to put a dislocated finger back into place.

FINGER TENDON INJURY

If your finger dangles from the end or middle joint and you can only straighten it by propping it up with the opposite hand, you probably have a tendon injury. This can happen when you bang your straightened-out finger on something. (When you can't straighten the joint even by using the other hand, there could be a break or dislocation.)

If you suspect a tendon injury and you can't see a health care provider, splint the joint and don't let it droop, even if you change splints. For an injured end joint, splint eight weeks. For an injured middle joint, splint six weeks. The tendon may heal, but often surgery is necessary. If you don't get surgery within three weeks of a middle-joint tendon injury, the odds of the bend remaining permanent are high.

✚ HOW TO AVOID A PERMANENTLY STIFF JOINT AFTER SPLINTING

When I was in medical school, I openly dislocated my index finger's middle joint while playing touch football. ("Openly" means the bone was exposed.) I had to wear a splint for six weeks. Try performing surgery while wearing one of those!

When I tried to flex my finger after the splint was off, the joint didn't budge. But after a few days of trying and trying, it creaked a little. I'm happy to say that thanks to persistence it now works as well as my other fingers. Now that I'm older I'm sure it would take even a lot more effort to get it working. But the alternative is a permanently stiff joint.

If you splint any joint for more than a few days, it's going to get stiff. The longer it's splinted, the harder it is to get it to loosen back up. If you want any chance of getting the joint working again, you need to diligently start loosening it as soon after splinting as you can. But forcing it could cause more damage. So use only the muscles that flex that joint.

For example, if you injure your finger, don't use the other hand to help loosen the joint. Instead, try to grip a ball. Initially you'll get only a tiny bit of movement, but with persistence, you'll see steady improvement.

PELVIC FRACTURE

A hard fall or any sort of trauma that carries a high-energy force, such as a car accident, can cause a pelvic fracture. On the other hand, a person with osteoporosis can break her pelvis while just standing.

Suspect a pelvic fracture after an injury if it hurts in that area while standing or when applying pressure. Initial treatment is a wide, tight band around the pelvis to keep the broken bones from moving. Clothing or a sleeping bag will do. There should be no bearing weight on the pelvis: at the very least, that means using crutches, but if the fracture could be unstable, the victim shouldn't stand. If you need to move her, a spinal board should be used (see page 63).

In high-force trauma, internal bleeding should be suspected (see page 167).

To check for an unstable or displaced pelvic fracture, examine the protrusions of the pelvic bones—you may call them hip bones. They're the ones you can feel on either side of your lower abdomen just below the ribs.

Suspect a displaced fracture if these bones are uneven while the victim is lying flat on her back. If they're equal, check them further: kneel, place a hand on each one, and press downward with equal force. If one moves, suspect an unstable fracture that may not be displaced but is at risk of becoming so.

A displaced or unstable fracture greatly increases the odds that the initial injury caused internal damage and the victim needs expert help as soon as possible. Meantime, she should be splinted and restrained with a spinal board. Moving her without a spinal board could cause additional injury to the pelvic organs and blood vessels.

HIP AND THIGH FRACTURES

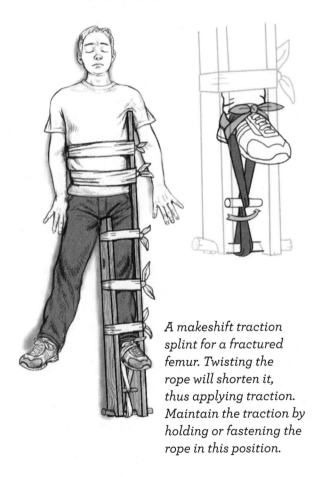

A makeshift traction splint for a fractured femur. Twisting the rope will shorten it, thus applying traction. Maintain the traction by holding or fastening the rope in this position.

Hip and thigh (femur) fractures usually result from falls or automobile accidents. Everything from just below the knee to just above the hip has to be splinted. There are special commercial splints for this, but in a pinch, you'll have to make do with what you have. And there should be no weight bearing on the leg at all.

A major concern is blood loss. If the middle of the bone is broken, the broken ends could damage the nearby large femoral artery, and there could be major blood loss into the thigh without much swelling. For this reason, seek immediate medical attention—including evacuation if you're in a remote area—for this type of fracture.

If that's not possible, apply traction by pulling on the lower leg. Make sure the pull is in line with the rest of the leg. This stretches the thigh muscles, tensing them around the break, and compresses the artery, which slows or stops the bleeding. And you'll need to find a way to continue the traction. The illustration on page 57 shows one way to do this. Most emergency professionals have a commercial device for this, which of course is a lot easier than trying to make your own contraption.

KNEE INJURIES

Sometimes just a little movement that twists your knee the wrong way tears the joint's cartilage or ligaments. Often you feel or hear a pop followed by pain.

One of the keys to initial treatment is keeping the joint stable. If you can move your knee in ways you shouldn't be able to, if you have pain, or if the knee feels unstable when walking, splint it. The splint should be long enough to be taped or wrapped to the thigh and lower leg while keeping the knee straight.

Get your weight off of the knee by lying down or sitting with the leg elevated, or use crutches.

If the knee is actually dislocated, this is an emergency because of possible injury to the nerves and arteries. A dislocated knee will be obvious when you compare it to the uninjured one. The upper and lower leg bones will not be anywhere close to aligned.

It is essential for a knee joint to be put back in place within the first few hours, or loss of the leg is likely. The way to do this is to pull on the lower leg with traction, but some knee dislocations are difficult to fix. Sometimes a dislocated knee goes back into place by itself, but it's still a serious injury and should be splinted. Even if the joint goes back into place, the nerves and arteries have more than likely been injured and loss of the lower leg is a major possibility. Get medical help as quickly as possible.

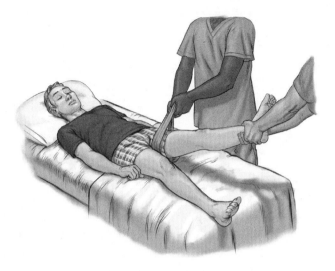

Pulling on the lower leg with traction.

KNEECAP DISLOCATION

The kneecap sits in a groove in the femur (thighbone) and glides back and forth smoothly. A twist or direct hit can knock it out of the groove, resulting in a bent knee with the kneecap more on the side than it should be. (Note that this is different from a knee dislocation, in which the entire joint is out of place.)

Usually, this can be resolved by slowly straightening out the leg, which lessens the tension on the muscles and ligaments holding the kneecap. At the same time, gently push on the kneecap to tease it back in place.

The knee needs to be splinted for about four weeks with the leg straight, and crutches should be used for about a week.

TIBIA OR FIBULA FRACTURE (LOWER LEG)

Of the two bones in the lower leg, the tibia (the bigger one—the shin) supports all the weight, so if it's broken, weight bearing—especially without splinting—can make for a catastrophe. If only the fibula is broken, you can usually get by with a little weight bearing since the tibia actually serves as a splint for the injury. You can get a clue to whether your tibia is broken by pressing along it—from its head (just below your knee) to the bottom of it (your ankle). If you find a tender place directly on the bone, there's likely a break there.

Whether or not the tibia is the bone that's broken, splint your leg for stability and use crutches. If the leg is crooked and help is not coming, you could try to apply traction by pulling on the ankle.

> ### Homemade Crutches
>
> Make crutches out of broomsticks, mops, or, even better, push brooms turned upside down. But be sure the tips are nonslip: cover them with cloth or, preferably, rubber.

ANKLE FRACTURE OR SPRAIN

An ankle injury is usually caused by twisting the ankle while standing, walking, running, or jumping. It's hard to tell a fracture from a sprain without an X-ray, but the initial treatment is the same. Use a splint and an elastic bandage, along with a cane or crutches. If there's no splint, wrap a bandage in a figure-of-eight method.

Any ankle injury is going to take four to six weeks to heal, on average. After that, the ankle joint will be weak and easy to retwist for a while, so consider keeping the elastic bandage on or wearing high-top boots, especially when walking on uneven ground.

FOOT FRACTURE

You can fracture your foot even without an obvious injury. In fact, you can develop a stress fracture simply by walking too much.

Without medical help, there's not a lot to do for this except wear a hard-sole shoe or boot and use a cane for about four weeks.

SPINE INJURY

Whenever someone has a head, neck, or back injury, you should suspect a spine injury. Whenever someone falls more than a few feet, even if he lands on his feet, you must suspect a spine injury. There's more. If no one saw the accident and the victim is unconscious—or even the least bit disoriented—and there's even a remote possibility that there could be a head or neck injury, you need to treat the victim as if he has sustained one.

In other words, this is a case of assuming guilt until innocence is proved. Unless you're sure there was no spine injury, you must assume there was one. That means not moving the victim—not even allowing her to slightly move her head—until you have either (1) ruled out a spine injury or (2) stabilized the spine so it will not move.

The reason to be so careful is simple. If part of a fractured vertebra moves and presses on the spinal cord, this could result in paralysis.

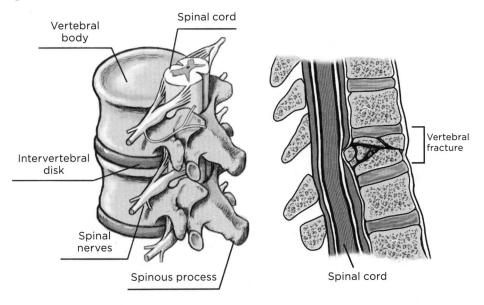

The vertebrae protect the spinal cord. The illustration on the right shows one type of vertebral fracture.

EXCEPTIONS TO THE RULE

If there's immediate, impending danger—for instance, if the victim is in the direct path of a forest fire or an oncoming train or unstable overhead rocks—you might have to make a judgment call and skip the no-movement rule. Even then, try to pad the neck if you have time, and move the victim as carefully as possible. One way to do this is with a trap squeeze (see page 66).

Another judgment-call situation is when there's serious bleeding, cardiac arrest, or another immediately life-threatening problem. It just makes sense to give priority to that before dealing with the spine. Even then, be as careful as you can.

HOW TO CHECK FOR A SPINE INJURY

To check a spine properly, it helps to have some training. A hands-on course is best.

Defer to expert medical assistance if at all possible, but if none is coming and the victim is alert, oriented, and cooperative, with no other painful, distracting injuries, assess the spine by following the steps below. (If the victim isn't alert, oriented, or cooperative or is distracted, skip this assessment and go to "Moving, Step 1" (page 63).)

1. **Ask for permission:** Consent is always a must before examining or treating anyone alert enough to reply.

2. **Slip a cervical collar on the victim without moving his head:** Use a commercially manufactured cervical collar if you have one, but if you don't, improvise with whatever soft materials—such as cloths, pillows, and sleeping bags—you have on hand. Arrange enough of the padding around the victim's neck to prevent his head from moving in any direction—including tilting up and down. Wrap or tape everything in place snugly but not so tightly that you risk choking the victim or impairing breathing in any way. If no padding is available, or there's any possibility that the victim might move, have someone hold the head, or you can kneel and hold it between your knees. Bottom line: never move the head or body, even during the exam.

3. **Press on each vertebra to check for tenderness:** The vertebrae are those protrusions you can feel in your spine. Start at the upper neck and work down. If the victim is lying on his back, you may not be able to get to the thoracic (chest-level) vertebrae, so press on each rib instead. If a vertebra connected to a rib is injured, pressing on that rib will elicit pain.

4. **Check the fingers and toes for sensation:** Use a safety pin or your fingernail to lightly scratch one side, then the other, of both feet and hands (without breaking the skin). Ask the victim to tell you which hand or foot—and which side of it—you're scratching. Check every toe and finger. Compare the sensation in one hand to the sensation in the other.

5. **Check muscle strength:** Ask the victim to flex his ankle by pointing his toes up toward the body. Give the top of the foot a little resistance with your hand. Next have him point his toes in the opposite direction, again with a little resistance from you. Have him grip a couple of your fingers and squeeze. Finally, have him spread all his fingers apart. Gently try to squeeze them together. For each test, compare sides to assess strength.

If you find tenderness along the spine, loss of sensation, or muscle weakness, assume there may be a spine injury. If you cannot rule out a spine injury, medical help becomes essential, even if you have to get it there by helicopter.

MOVING, STEP 1: PREPARE A BACKBOARD

If you do have to move the victim, take a minute to assess the situation and make a plan. Try to gather some helpers—ideally, at least three. Then prepare a backboard.

1. If you have a commercial backboard, that's best. Otherwise, find a stiff board as long as or longer than the victim. Perhaps take a door off its hinges, remove the legs from a table, or, for a short victim, use an ironing board. If nothing else, bind together long, sturdy poles, but remember this: the backboard must be strong, straight, and so sturdy that there's no possibility of its breaking or bending even slightly. If there is, don't use it. On the other hand, if you and others have to move the victim very far, the more the board weighs, the more difficult moving him will be.

2. Next, find seven long strips of cloth or pieces of rope, which you'll use to tie the victim to the board. Place them under the board (see the illustration below for positioning). Make sure the strips are long enough to wrap around the victim and tie.

3. Slide the board next to the victim.

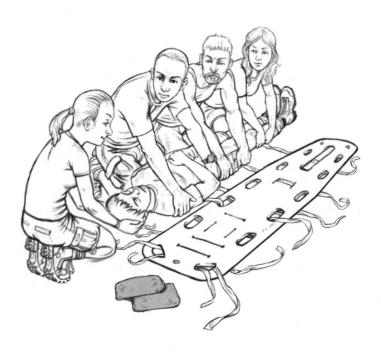

STICKS, STONES, AND BROKEN BONES

MOVING, STEP 2: PREPARE FOR THE LOGROLL

Logrolling is the most universally accepted way to properly move someone onto a backboard. It's also the best method for moving someone onto his side to help his breathing. The goal is to avoid twisting or flexing the spine at all—keeping it as straight as if the victim were a board.

The logrolling process should have a leader. Let's assume it's you. Before the roll, have everyone and everything ready.

1. **Get yourself into position:** Kneel above the victim's head and keep it still. During the roll, you'll be in charge of rolling the head at the same speed as the body, making sure the neck doesn't rotate. If the victim is lying on his back, you may be able to kneel down and hold his head between your knees until you're ready to do the roll. If you're alone, you may have to hold the victim's head and have him try to assist you with the move, but this is far from ideal.

2. **Get the other helpers into position:** Have your helpers kneel beside the victim's body, which should be between them and the backboard. They'll be reaching over to grab the side of the victim closer to the backboard, then rolling him toward them so the backboard can be scooted directly behind him. If there's only you and one other person, that person should kneel with one hand on the victim's opposite shoulder and one on his hip. If there's a second helper, that person should kneel and have one hand on the victim's hip and the other on his leg. A third helper should be responsible for the knees and for repositioning the board when needed.

3. **Get the victim into position:** There are two lines of thought about what to do at this point if the victim isn't conveniently already lying in a perfectly straight line. You could keep the person in whatever position you've found him and perhaps position him more neutrally during the logroll or just after. Or, before the roll, you could go ahead and put the person in what's called the neutral position: gently turn the head, shoulders, hips, and legs so they're straight, parallel, and facing the same way. Either way, any movement of the spine is a risk, but somehow you have to roll the victim to get him onto the board.

MOVING, STEP 3: PERFORM THE LOGROLL

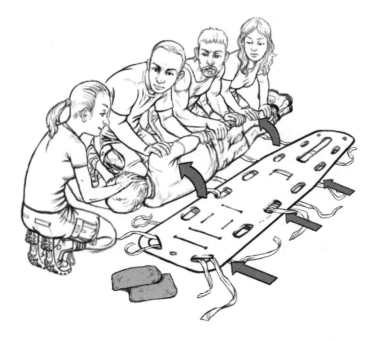

As the leader, make sure everyone knows what to do before you start. Then:

1. Have everyone pull the victim on his side in unison on the count of three.

2. Have a helper slide the board as close as she can get it to the victim's back.

3. Have everyone, on the count of three, logroll the body back onto the board.

MOVING, STEP 4: SECURE THE VICTIM

Now you'll secure the victim to the backboard. This is to make sure his spine doesn't move during transport and he doesn't fall off the board.

1. Have someone hold the victim's head in place throughout this process.

2. Stabilize the back and neck. Stuff anything soft in every space, nook, and cranny around and under the back and neck, still without moving the spine. You might also put something under the knees so they can be flexed a little for comfort. Stuff everything in so tightly that nothing can possibly move when you pick the board up and start the transport. Firm foam is a good choice, or roll up towels, blankets, sleeping bags, or a tarp. Clothing is another option. Make sure nothing is impairing breathing.

3. Cover the victim to prevent hypothermia.

4. Tie the victim securely to the board using the ropes or cloths that you previously placed underneath it. (If you see a place you think the rope might rub raw, place a little padding between the rope and the skin.) Start with the ties at the lower legs, thighs, and hips. Crisscross the two ropes at the upper chest. Each should go over one shoulder and under the opposite arm. Tie the head down last, around the chin and around the forehead.

Make sure the body is secure enough to stay still even if the board tilts a bit. Periodically check the chest, neck, and head to make sure nothing is impairing breathing.

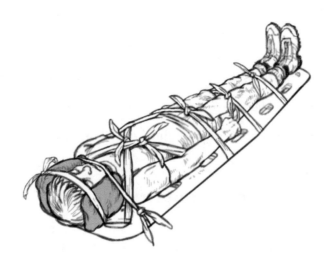

OPTIONAL MOVEMENT MANEUVER: TRAP SQUEEZE

If you have no one to help you do the logroll, or if you need to quickly move a victim over a short distance to get him out of danger, you can squat at his head, grab the shoulder muscles on both sides of the neck (the trapezius muscles, or traps), squeeze the head with your arms to stabilize it, and pull the person. Try not to raise the head any more than you have to, and pull in a straight line so there's no twisting. You can also pull a victim onto a backboard this way by placing the foot of the board at his head and pulling him onto it lengthwise.

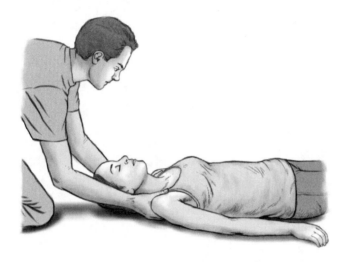

4

ALTERED STATES

POP QUIZ

A woman came home to find her fifty-two-year-old husband lying on the floor. She called his name, and he sat up but otherwise didn't acknowledge her. When she tried to help him get up, he fought and pushed her away, still staring straight ahead, not talking. He had no known health problems and didn't drink alcohol or take drugs—at least not to her knowledge. She called 911. But what if she couldn't have? What should she have done first?

A. Scanned her surroundings for clues to his condition and potential dangers.

B. Looked for evidence of alcohol or drugs.

C. Tried her best to get him to a chair.

D. Opened the windows or gotten him outside.

ANSWERS

A. Correct. Any time you come upon someone who appears sick or injured, take a quick scan of the surroundings, looking for clues, and to make sure that whatever might have affected the victim (intruder, wild animal, falling rocks) isn't a danger to you, too. In this case, the woman should look for evidence of a struggle or forced entry. If there is, perhaps she could yell for help, get something to use as a club, or at least be prepared to run.

B. Incorrect. This is the second step to take. Don't assume that drugs or alcohol weren't involved. Go through the AEIOU TIPS acronym (see page 72) to consider likely causes of altered consciousness and what to do for them.

C. Incorrect. The woman shouldn't move the victim at all until she's done a quick check for head, neck, or back trauma. After that, there's no hurry to get him into a chair. He's better off on the floor in case he faints. And he's somewhat combative, so there's no reason to provoke him.

D. Incorrect. Unless you suspect carbon monoxide could be the problem. Especially in the winter, carbon monoxide—a colorless, odorless, and deadly gas—is a danger. It's produced by burning all sorts of things and can come from a gas leak in the house. If your quick scan of the surroundings (in answer A) leads you to think carbon monoxide might be the issue, getting the victim outside is a priority.

In a few hours, this man came back to his old self and had no idea what had caused his problem. All his tests came back negative. It was thought that he may have had a seizure, but there was no evidence that he'd bitten his tongue (see page 73), his seizure tests were negative, and he's lived into his eighties without a recurrence. Sometimes watchful waiting can be the best medicine

DIAGNOSING ALTERED MENTAL STATUS

Altered mental status could mean anything from a little disorientation to complete unconsciousness. Something that has adversely affected the brain isn't allowing the victim to think as he normally would. The challenge is figuring out the cause: you can't rely on the victim to tell you what happened. So it's detective time.

HOW TO RECOGNIZE ALTERED MENTAL STATUS

If a person is unconscious or is acting inappropriately—maybe acting like someone who's had a bit too much to drink—an altered mental status is obvious. But sometimes the clues can be more subtle and are likely to be missed unless you test for them. Do a screening exam whenever there's a possibility of head injury or serious trauma—or if your suspicions are raised, even a little. The exam, called an alertness and orientation check, is quick and easy, and the results may surprise you.

Step 1: Alertness Check

First note the victim's alertness level. Is he anxious, groggy, or hard to wake up? Many emergency personnel use the acronym AVPU as a memory jog for evaluating alertness. With this acronym, they can communicate status to each other and also monitor whether the person's getting better. Each letter corresponds to a level of alertness, going from better to worse.

Alert: The victim is awake and responds appropriately to questions and directions. (If the victim passes this level, this doesn't mean there's no altered mental status. Go to step 2—the orientation check—to make sure he's completely alert.)

Voice: The victim is not alert but will acknowledge questions or commands, even if it's with a mumble.

Pain: The victim won't respond to voice commands but will respond to pain—i.e., he might grimace if pinched.

Unresponsive: The victim won't respond to anything.

If the victim is alert, it's time to get more detailed with an orientation check.

Step 2: Orientation Check

The orientation check takes some cooperation and may require insistence on your part. The victim may be in pain or anxious and really not interested in answering your questions unless you can convince him that he must do so in order for you to help him. If he steadfastly refuses, that tells you you're not going to be able to rely on his responses. On the other hand, even if the testing is normal, you'll have a baseline to refer to in case something changes.

The four general questions to ask during the orientation check can be thought of as who, what, where, and when—otherwise known as person, event, place, and time. Ask the questions periodically to see if there's been a change. If the initial checks are abnormal, if there's been trauma, or if you're really worried for whatever reason, you might check every fifteen minutes or so. If the results get worse, do a reassessment for causes you may have missed. (Of course, if the victim's condition worsens, that's all the more reason to try to get expert care as soon as possible.) If the results get better or at least don't get worse, you may want to extend the time between testing to thirty minutes, then an hour, then longer.

- **Person:** Ask, "Who are you?" Insist that the victim give you his name. If you don't know him, ask a friend or relative for verification or check his ID, if has one with him. If he knows you, ask, "Do you know who I am?" If he says yes, ask, "What's my name?" Or ask, "Is this your friend? What's her name?"

- **Event:** Ask, "What happened?" There's no need to go into specifics. But he should know the basics—that he was hit in the head, fell, took medicine, had been drinking, has diabetes, or whatever the case might be.

- **Place:** Ask, "Where are you?" Again, a general answer—such as "In the park," "At home," or "In [the name of the city]"—will do.

- **Time:** Ask, "What day is it?" Or at least, "What month is it?" or "What year is it?"

If he gets any of the answers wrong, he has an altered mental status. If you're not sure of the cause, it's time to start looking.

✚ HOW TO KEEP THE VICTIM FROM CHOKING

When someone with an altered mental status isn't fully awake and is lying on his back, he could easily get vomit or a lot of saliva into his lungs. So prop him on his side to prevent this. If there's any possibility at all of a spine injury, use the logroll method on page 64.

COMMON CAUSES

The reason for altered mental status determines what should be done next. If the cause is not apparent, you may find clues while performing a quick physical exam.

It helps to know some of the causes and clues you'll be looking for. The mnemonic AEIOU TIPS won't cover every one of them, but it's a way to jog your memory on many of the more common ones. (Some letters in this mnemonic can refer to more than one type of condition. Perhaps a better mnemonic would be AEIOU TTIPPS? An altered version for altered status?) Unless you're absolutely certain of the reason, be a good detective and never make your final conclusion until you've finished the entire exam. There can be more than one cause, or there can be a contributing factor outside of the AEIOU TIPS.

Alcohol

Clues: The odor of alcohol; liquor bottles.

Treatment: If alcohol is the only reason for an altered mental status, the only treatment in the field is just to hope the victim can safely sleep it off. Be sure he's on his side in case he vomits—and to keep his airway open. And remember: just because a victim has alcohol on his breath doesn't mean there's not another reason for the altered state.

Epilepsy (Seizure)

Clues: A medical alert bracelet or a card in the wallet. There are often bite marks on the tongue.

Treatment: See page 77.

Infection

Clues: Signs of illness before the mental status became altered (though there often aren't any). Confusion in an elderly person can be the first sign of something as simple as a bladder infection. Fever is another clue, but even if it's high, the skin can be cool and clammy—and the skin can be flushed and warm without fever.

Treatment: Depends on the infection type and severity. Quick diagnosis and treatment improves the chance of survival, so it's essential to get expert care as soon as possible.

Overdose

Clues: Pill bottles; needle marks. Pinpoint pupils are a sign of opiate overdose— heroin, morphine, codeine, or certain other pain medicines. Large, dilated pupils are a clue that cocaine or sedatives might have been the cause.

Treatment: For a suspected opiate overdose, the drug naloxone now comes in a prefilled autoinjector and in a nasal inhaler. Some homeless shelters and family members of drug abusers may have it. Of course, a person can overdose on any medicine. The national poison control center's number is 1-800-222-2222.

Uremia

Uremia is a buildup of toxins in the blood that happens when the kidneys aren't working properly to flush them out.

Clues: A medical alert bracelet or wallet card; known kidney problems. People with chronic renal failure who have to get dialysis (an artificial way to flush the toxins) may have a large, firm tube implanted in an arm to provide easy needle access to a vein. Blood can be felt flowing through it.

Treatment: Barring expert dialysis, you can only treat a reversible underlying cause (such as poison, infection, or dehydration), if there is one, and hope the kidneys start refunctioning.

Trauma or Temperature

Clues to trauma: Evidence from a physical examination (see page 76) or finding the victim in a situation that indicates possible injury. Treatment depends on the nature of the trauma.

Clues to temperature: Evidence of hypothermia or hyperthermia (see page 232–237 for treatment options).

Insulin

We're talking diabetes here—the underlying problem being either too little or too much insulin. A person can have too much insulin (low blood sugar) if he's injected himself with the wrong quantity, and he can have too little insulin (high blood sugar) if he's forgotten to take his medication.

Clues: A medical alert bracelet or wallet card; some people might even have an insulin pump strapped to their bodies or their clothes that's connected to an IV-type tube, which in turn is connected to a needle that's inserted in the skin. Many a police officer (and doctor) has been fooled initially into thinking that a serious diabetic condition is nothing more than alcohol overindulgence, since both can cause agitation.

Treatment: Give the victim a little food or fruit juice. This increases blood sugar levels, helping someone with low blood sugar recover. It won't help people with high blood sugar, but it's unlikely to harm them. Unless you're specially trained on properly giving insulin, there's nothing to do in the field for someone with high blood sugar. (Never give anything orally unless you're sure the victim is alert enough to swallow it. An option is to rub a little sugar, or the closest thing you have to something sweet, into the victim's gums. Just beware of teeth and make sure the substance is nothing the victim could suck into his lungs.) If you're lucky, an insulin-dependent diabetic might have a glucagon emergency kit. Glucagon is a hormone that can be injected to raise the blood sugar.

Poison or Psychiatric Illness

Clues to poison: Bottles; bad food; knowing the victim has eaten a plant.

Treatment for poison: Many times, as with alcohol overdose (see page 73), all you can do is try to keep the person's airway open and give time for the poison to wear off. Some poisons have antidotes, and that's one of the reasons to call the national poison control center (1-800-222-2222) and 911 if you can. Never induce vomiting in someone who's drowsy or lethargic; he could get vomit in his lungs (see page 77).

Clues to psychiatric illness: Prescription bottles of psychiatric medications or a known history of mental illness. The person may be acting strange, hallucinating, or be extremely agitated.

Treatment: This can be complicated. Options include giving the person his medication if he needs it and trying to calm him down—or at least not excite him more. In the worst cases, you may need to remove yourself from the situation for your own safety.

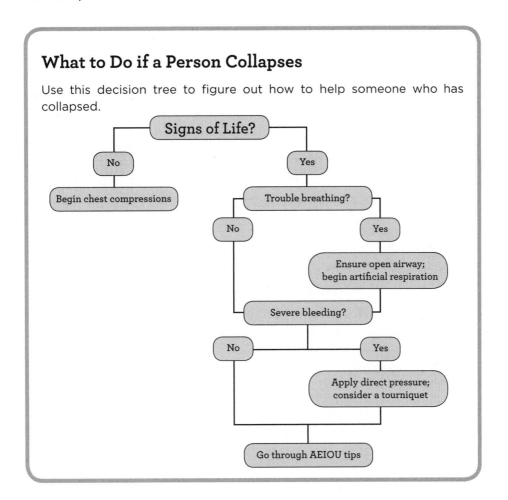

What to Do if a Person Collapses

Use this decision tree to figure out how to help someone who has collapsed.

Signs of Life?

No → Begin chest compressions

Yes → Trouble breathing?

No →

Yes → Ensure open airway; begin artificial respiration

Severe bleeding?

No →

Yes → Apply direct pressure; consider a tourniquet

Go through AEIOU tips

Stroke

Clues: Facial drooping; arm or leg weakness on one side; garbled, slurred, or non-sensical speech.

Treatment: See page 80.

THE ALTERED MENTAL STATUS PHYSICAL EXAM

No matter what you think the cause of an altered mental status is, if the victim is unconscious or doesn't pass all four parts of the orientation exam (person, event, place, and time), it's time to do a physical exam.

If you're dealing with an unresponsive, unconscious person, always start by checking for signs of life, such as breathing. If you find none, start chest compressions (see page 141). Also immediately stop any profuse bleeding. Continue chest compressions until expert help arrives or you're exhausted.

For someone who has signs of life or who's conscious, you can do a more detailed exam. While performing it, if there's any chance that the spine could have been injured, or if you don't know what happened, do not move or twist any part of the spine, including the neck. Movement can cause paralysis if any of the vertebrae are fractured.

If you have a partner, she can hold the victim's head steady during the exam. If he's lying down, have your partner kneel above his head and hold it between her hands.

Before beginning the exam, if the victim is awake, ask for his permission to touch him before performing any physical exam. If he says yes, consider doing the following:

1. Treat any wounds that are profusely bleeding by applying direct pressure or a tourniquet. Do this before performing the rest of the exam. This step alone could save a life.

2. Feel the head for swollen spots. If there are depressions in the skull that could be fractures, don't try to manipulate them. Doing so without specialized equipment is much more likely to cause harm than good. Just protect the area as best you can.

3. Quickly check the rest of the body for evidence of trauma.

4. Check purses and wallets for any clues to medical problems. Also check for a medical bracelet.

5. Examine the eyes and ears. Two black eyes (called raccoon eyes) or bruises behind the ears without evidence of direct trauma to these areas can be a sign of internal bleeding. A continuous dripping of blood from an ear or nostril,

again without direct trauma, can indicate severe head injury. So can clear fluid from an ear or nostril. Any of these signs means expert help is needed quickly if possible, because there's not much to do for these problems outside of a hospital.

6. Check the tongue for bite marks (common during seizures).

7. Open the eyelids to make sure the pupils are the same size. If you have a light, shine it in one eye to see if the pupil constricts, then shine it in the other eye. Normal pupils don't rule out anything, but unequal pupil sizes or a difference in how one side reacts to light can be a sign of bleeding or swelling in the brain. Expert help is needed ASAP.

HOW TO CHECK THE PUPILS

Checking the pupils can be a little trickier than you might imagine. For one thing, don't get too hung up on slight differences in size and reaction time. It'll drive you crazy.

1. Look in the eyes and compare to make sure the pupils are equal.

2. If you have a flashlight, shine it in one eye, then quickly move the light away. The pupil should constrict with the light, then dilate when the light is moved. Do the same to the other eye and compare. The time it takes each to constrict should be same.

If the surroundings are pretty bright, first cover both eyes to allow the pupils to dilate. (Covering just one eye wouldn't work; both pupils would still stay constricted because they typically constrict or dilate together.) Quickly uncover one eye and watch for constriction. Do this several times if you need to.

TREATMENT

Whatever the cause, there are some general things you can do for most people who have an altered mental status:

1. Ensure an open airway. If the victim is lying down and not fully awake, turning him on his side will help the tongue stay clear of the back of the throat and will help any fluids, such as saliva or vomit, run out of the mouth and not down the windpipe. Unless you're absolutely sure that head or neck trauma was not involved, you should only move a person using the logroll technique (see page 64).

2. **If you suspect the underlying cause, treat it.** Give insulin or food, give antibiotics, stop the bleeding, and so on.

3. **Cover the victim.** Hypothermia is a frequently forgotten risk, and it can happen in temperatures well above freezing.

4. **Let the victim sleep.** If he is somewhat alert, sooner or later he's going to want to sleep. That's normal. Just make sure he continues to breathe without difficulty. Every hour or two, you can wake him to check his pupils and ask the orientation questions. But after a night or two, that's going to get old. Consider gradually lengthening the times between checks, unless the evaluation suggests the victim is getting worse and therefore changes your treatment or evacuation plan. Letting him sleep can be healing.

CONCUSSION

Entire books could be written about concussion—and several have been—but in general, two things must be present for a diagnosis of concussion: (1) the victim must have had some sort of head trauma, either from a direct blow or from something that's caused the head to violently jerk, and (2) there must be a symptom or symptoms caused by the injury other than a tender spot in the bone or tissue where the trauma occurred. The symptoms can range from loss of consciousness to being dazed to just seeing stars after the trauma. The victim might have a bad headache, double or blurred vision, nausea, vomiting, or dizziness. Or the symptom could be more along the lines of amnesia, trouble sleeping, or a decreased ability to concentrate. Basically, we're looking for any symptom that could have resulted from a bruise to the brain.

TREATMENT

For as long as there are any symptoms, the basic treatment is rest, physically and mentally. Despite popular belief, it's okay to let someone with a concussion sleep. However, at least until the victim seems to be getting better, someone should check on him every few hours to make sure the symptoms aren't worsening. No reading, no computer work, no watching television or listening to the radio. It doesn't have to be complete bed rest, but not resting at all can prolong the symptoms quite a bit. Even when the symptoms are gone, only gradually increase activity. If the symptoms start up again, the victim should stop whatever activity is causing them until he feels okay again. Even then, he should consider resting an extra day or two before trying the activity again.

By the way, anyone involved in coaching or managing a sports team, no matter the age of the participants, is likely to have some training in recognizing and dealing with concussions.

RED FLAGS

Anyone with a concussion should be checked by a health care professional if at all possible. If you're the one with the injury, don't rely solely on your own assessment for signs you're getting worse and need reevaluation. Instead, someone you trust should be keeping an eye out for any changes in your condition.

To ferret out some of the clues that there could be serious damage from head trauma needing immediate expert care, remember your ABCDEFS:

- **Alert:** If the victim is not alert and fully oriented within at least thirty minutes after the trauma, that's a big concern.

- **Blood:** If there's blood dripping from an ear, unless you're sure it's from a direct injury to the ear, it could be from a serious skull fracture that has damaged a blood vessel or even the lining around the brain.

- **Conscious:** Any loss of consciousness is a concern, but one that lasts more than a couple of minutes is especially worrisome.

- **Diffuse (all-over) headache:** If there's not just pain in the area of the injury but also severe pain that is deep and spread throughout the head, and if it isn't getting a lot better with time or something like acetaminophen (Tylenol), that's a sign of possible serious damage. Because it increases the risk of internal bleeding, the victim shouldn't take aspirin. Even an NSAID such as ibuprofen might slightly increase the risk. And if the victim takes a narcotic you won't know if it's the medicine or the trauma causing a change in her mental status and pupils. So until the victim has been thoroughly checked by an expert and told that these medicines are okay to take, she should avoid them.

- **Eyes:** If your pupils are normal, it doesn't mean you don't have a serious head injury. But if they're clearly unequal or don't constrict equally to light, that could be a sign of expanding pressure on the brain, and this condition requires immediate attention. Just try to make sure the pupil wasn't already like that before the injury—perhaps because of a prior problem or even because one of the eyes is artificial. Yes, I've seen it happen.

- **Fluid:** Fluid flowing from the nostrils or ears, especially if it's clear, could be from a tear in the lining around the brain that holds in the cerebrospinal fluid.

- **Seizure:** A seizure after head trauma can be a sign that there's been a serious brain injury.

STROKE

A stroke can happen at any age. I know a person who had one in his midthirties. Several stroke-awareness groups currently tout the mnemonic FAST to remind you of common symptoms. That's facial drooping (on one side), arm weakness (in one arm—or even weakness in one leg), or speech difficulty. The T stands for time to call 911.

You can check for facial drooping by asking the victim to show you his teeth; then ask him to close his eyes tightly. Check for one-sided muscle weakness by having him grip your fingers with each of his hands. Listen for slurred speech by asking him to repeat a simple sentence.

Treatments can sometimes reverse the damage from strokes or at least limit further progression, but they can only be done in a medical facility such as a hospital emergency room and are most likely to help if they're started quickly.

If expert treatment is unavailable, you'll just have to keep the victim at rest (it's safest to have him lie down; just make sure the airway stays open; see page 157) and warm. Give fluids and food if he can ingest them without choking. Giving an aspirin is risky, because some strokes are caused by bleeding blood vessels.

Keep in mind that even with limited care, a stroke is not always a death sentence. With time, some stroke victims may become more alert and active. Predicting who survives, who ends up with debilitating permanent problems, and who dies can be difficult. A longer recovery process, however, usually makes for a graver prognosis.

SEIZURE

Also called convulsions, a seizure is an abnormal conduction of electrical transmissions in the brain. It doesn't always involve severe jerking, the classic symptom people associate with it. Sometimes the victim just falls to the ground, her muscles stiff. In one particular type of seizure the only sign may be a sudden, unresponsive staring into space, sometimes with frequent blinking or smacking of the lips. It's common for a seizure to last up to a couple of minutes. Maybe even three.

Other signs that someone's had a seizure are:

• Urinary incontinence during the seizure

• A fairly prolonged period of grogginess and confusion after the seizure has subsided. It may take minutes to hours for full alertness to return. If a victim isn't sure what happened but can recall being confused for a minute or more, a seizure should be suspected. Confusion from fainting, on the other hand, rarely lasts more than thirty seconds.

• Evidence that the victim bit her tongue during the seizure

• A medical alert bracelet

CAUSES

Potential causes of seizures include:

• Epilepsy, a disease that is treatable with prescription medicine

• A recent brain injury

• An infection, such as the onset of meningitis or encephalitis

• Low sodium, magnesium, or glucose in the blood

• Drugs, such as cocaine

• Withdrawal from alcohol in someone who's been drinking heavily for several days or longer

ALTERED STATES

TREATMENT

During the seizure, do nothing other than make sure the victim doesn't hurt herself. Ensure that no potentially injury-causing objects are in the way. Never stick anything in the person's mouth. You're much more likely to cause harm than good. There may be a period of deep sleep after the seizure. If there's any trouble breathing, gently turn the person onto her side. (If there's any possibility of spine injury, see page 64.)

If there's no medical bracelet indicating the victim has epilepsy and no one knows whether she has a history of seizures, try to get immediate expert care if possible if (1) the seizure lasts over three minutes or (2) another seizure occurs soon after the first. Either of these things puts the person at a high risk for permanent brain damage or even death. To try to get a seizure like this to stop, an intravenous antiseizure medicine or sedative such as benzodiazepine or lorazepam can be injected into a vein. Some seizure patients might have a rectal or dissolvable (oral) form on hand for emergencies. Occasionally a carotid massage of the type used for paroxysmal supraventricular tachycardia (PSVT; see page 134) may work to stop the seizure. Also, remember to do what you can to keep the airway open (see page 157).

After either a short or long seizure, when the grogginess and confusion wear off, you should be able to find out from the victim whether seizures are a known problem and if something is out of the ordinary regarding this particular episode. But be patient. It's not uncommon for someone getting over a seizure to be quite irritated.

FAINTING

Fainting—the medical term is syncope—is a sudden and temporary loss of consciousness caused by lack of adequate blood flow to the brain. That's different from getting knocked out or losing consciousness from, say, a drug overdose or an insulin coma.

True story: in my first year of medical school, we were all standing in a lab room and were told to partner up and prick each other's fingers with a sterile lancet. I heard a crash across the room. One of my classmates had fainted.

By the time I saw what was going on, he was getting up. He finished the test, and last I heard, he was a successful surgeon.

Over the years, I've instituted a rule: no matter how tough someone with an injury appears, I have him or her sit or lie down. And anyone who's with the injured person must sit down also. Many people faint if they remain standing, especially if there's blood and they try to watch the treatment procedure.

WARNING SIGNS OF FAINTING

In addition to the usual lightheadedness, people who faint often have other warning signs:

- Nausea
- Sweating
- Fast, shallow breathing
- Tunnel vision
- Clamminess
- Paleness
- Dizziness

TYPES OF FAINTING

Before learning what to do for someone who's fainted, it's helpful to learn some of the reasons for fainting. Dehydration and heart problems, for example, are two potential causes, and they require different treatments.

In a survival situation you may not always know the reason for fainting, but you can at least be aware of some causes and what you can and can't do about them. Here are some of the most common. Depending on what sources you read, the names and how the causes are classified vary, so focus on the causes and name them what you like.

Vasovagal Syncope: When Healthy People Faint

Vasovagal syncope, which involves the vagus nerve, is the most common type of fainting. Fright, pain, anxiety, and fast breathing can bring this on. Sometimes the trigger can be the sight of blood; sometimes it's coughing; urinating; straining, as with a bowel movement or lifting something heavy; or even laughing. It's why my medical classmate passed out.

The vagus nerve starts in the brain stem and works its way down the side of the neck and into the chest and abdomen. One of its jobs is to help regulate your blood pressure. Vasovagal syncope happens when your vagus nerve reacts to a situation by suddenly lowering your blood pressure (through decreasing your heart rate, relaxing your arteries, or both). This results in a sudden lack of blood to the brain. The vasovagal reaction can also cause certain symptoms to precede the fainting, such as increased respirations, sweating, nausea, and a faster heartbeat. Why a particular situation will trigger that sort of reaction in some people and not others is poorly understood. It's also called reflex or situational syncope.

Postural Syncope: Standing Up and Falling Down

When you stand, your body has to react in a way that ensures that blood flow continues to the brain. For this, it needs a strong heart that's beating well, blood vessels that constrict when they're supposed to, and enough blood cells and fluid in the arteries. If the adjustment process takes longer than usual, a type of fainting called postural syncope may occur.

Blood loss, severe anemia, and dehydration can cause postural syncope. Also, standing in one spot too long can pool so much blood in the legs that the heart temporarily lacks an adequate supply to pump to the brain.

Another type of fainting-upon-standing is called orthostatic syncope. This one happens without any of the above causes—and it's an ongoing problem in people who have it. Their bodies' monitors don't work correctly, so the mechanisms that keep blood going to the brain when they stand up don't go into effect. Orthostatic syncope can cause disability and may need specific treatment. It's usually seen in elderly people but can also be caused by certain medications. In the latter case, the medication should be changed under the supervision of the prescriber.

Cardiac Syncope: When Your Heart Fails You

Heart problems, such as a heart attack or congestive heart failure, can lessen blood flow to the brain and cause fainting. Other cardiac conditions—for example, if the heart pauses too long or beats too fast or slow, or if the heart muscle is weakened—can also prevent the heart from delivering blood to the brain fast enough.

Neurological Syncope: Brain Drain

Rarely, a migraine can cause fainting, as can a transient ischemic attack (TIA), also known as a mini stroke or reversible stroke.

TREATMENT

No matter the cause, if someone suddenly appears sweaty or has a vacant look in her eyes, suggest she sit down and bend over so her head is lower than her chest. If she's willing, lying down is even better. If she starts to fall, try helping her down so she won't get hurt. (Don't hurt yourself in the process.) Never keep her upright, because this may continue to keep blood from getting to the brain.

Once the head is as low as or lower than the heart, the victim should regain consciousness, albeit probably in a groggy state. Have her stay in that position for several minutes until the symptoms subside. Check the pulse and blood pressure if you have a cuff. Make sure they're normal before she tries to get up. Then she can sit for a few minutes, and if there are no symptoms, she could slowly try to stand.

If the symptoms recur, help her lower herself again, let the symptoms subside, and slowly try once more.

If the person is able to sit up for a few minutes and eventually stand, the cause is likely vasovagal, especially if you can pinpoint a trigger, such as a fright or the sight of blood. If you're not sure it's vasovagal, call 911 if possible. Meanwhile, try to get a quick medical history and physical evaluation.

Often, the likely reason for the fainting is pretty obvious, like if the person has lost a lot of blood or is dehydrated from vomiting. Other times, a little detective work is required. Here are some of the red flags that indicate that something serious is going on and that expert treatment, if available, is a must:

- No warning signs before fainting, or heart palpitations that last more than a few seconds before the victim passes out: this means the heart could be to blame (see page 80) and needs immediate evaluation

- Passing out while exercising: although this may turn out to be vasovagal and not serious, it can also be the only sign of an otherwise asymptomatic heart problem, which would increase the risk of sudden death with exercise in the future

- Pupils that are unequal in size: this means there could be serious pressure on the brain from a stroke (see page 80), trauma, or a tumor

- A severe headache: this could indicate a migraine or stroke

- Double vision, which could mean stroke, migraine, or brain tumor

- Excruciating back or abdominal pain, which could be a sign of a dissecting aortic aneurysm, a condition in which the wall of the aorta—the blood vessel connected straight from the heart—starts tearing apart: immediate transfer to a hospital could mean the difference between life and death

SHOCK

"He's going into shock!" On TV, this popular line comes with frenzied activity, confused yelling, and furrowed brows. But in real life . . . well, yeah, shock is bad news.

When you go into shock, your entire body—all its organs and living tissue—isn't getting enough blood and, hence, oxygen. Oxygen-carrying blood can only travel through the body effectively if (1) the heart is strong enough to pump it properly, (2) the blood vessels are constricting and expanding correctly to keep the pressure and flow even, and (3) you have enough blood to fill the vessels. If you don't, your heart can compensate somewhat by increasing the rate of pumping, but there comes a point when that's not enough.

Shock is life-threatening. Though expert help is needed if possible, there are some things you can do for shock in the field.

WHAT SHOCK IS NOT

TV and movies get it wrong here, at least in medical terms. Someone does not go into physical shock because of some sudden, severe psychological stress. Sure, a person can faint or become unfocused, detached, and confused, and that is serious. But it isn't in itself life-threatening and doesn't require the treatments detailed below. And yes, someone might have a heart attack from stress (after which he could go into cardiogenic shock), but in general, psychological or mental shock is altogether different from physical shock and treatment may just involve time or psychological therapies.

CLUES

Signs and symptoms of shock are:

- Cool, clammy skin
- Rapid, shallow breathing
- Rapid pulse
- Low blood pressure

- Confusion
- Difficulty staying awake
- Glazed eyes that aren't focusing

TREATMENT

For any type of shock, give fresh air at least. Supplemental oxygen is better. Have the victim lie down, and maintain an open airway (see page 157). Keep the victim warm with blankets unless hyperthermia is the problem. Generally, getting fluids into the system is a major priority unless internal bleeding or a weak heart is a possibility. If it is, the fluids must be given slowly, if at all.

When someone goes into shock, quickly getting expert treatment may be the only thing that saves the person's life, but here are some things you can try for various kinds of shock if you can't get medical help.

Hypovolemic Shock

Blood loss or dehydration can decrease the volume of fluid in the blood vessels past the point where the heart and remaining blood can compensate. Also, with blood loss, you have fewer red blood cells to carry the needed oxygen.

If the victim is alert, have her drink fluids. If intravenous fluids are given, they shouldn't be given too fast to anyone with underlying heart problems. They must also be given slowly to someone who might have internal bleeding, since too much pressure could break loose clots and aggravate the bleeding.

Blood transfusions may be needed.

Anaphylactic Shock

In anaphylactic shock, a severe allergic reaction produces chemicals that cause the lung airways to dangerously narrow and the blood vessels to expand when they should be constricting to keep blood pressure up. Injectable epinephrine (such as an EpiPen; see page 102) is the essential treatment for anaphylactic shock. People with severe allergies or asthma often keep this prescription device on hand for such an emergency. If that's not available, a prescribed albuterol inhaler (usually used for asthma) or prescribed steroids could be tried. Over-the-counter antihistamines (found in many allergy medicines) such as diphenhydramine (Benadryl) may also help. Chapter 5 has more information about anaphylaxis in the section about beestings (page 100). No matter the reason for the anaphylactic shock, the initial treatment is the same.

Cardiogenic Shock

A heart attack, congestive heart failure, an infection of the heart muscle, an abnormal heart rate, or a defective heart valve can weaken the heart's ability to pump blood. Severe hypothermia or hyperthermia could also weaken the heart.

Have the victim lie down, as you would for other types of shock, but in this case, the head should be elevated at least slightly to avoid fluid accumulation in the lungs.

For cardiogenic shock, specialized medicines not found outside a medical facility are usually essential, though if the problem is paroxysmal supraventricular tachycardia (PSVT), a carotid massage and other vagal maneuvers could be tried (see page 136).

Septic Shock

A severe infection can directly damage blood vessels or induce the body to produce chemicals that affect the vessels' ability to constrict when they need to. In this case, treatment is intravenous fluids, antibiotics, steroids, and other medicines. If an IV is impossible, give fluids by mouth if the victim is alert enough to drink without choking. If IV antibiotics are not an option, IM (intramuscular) injections would be the next best method of delivery, then oral antibiotics.

Neurogenic Shock

Nerves tell the blood vessels and heart what to do and when to do it. If the brain or nerves are damaged by, say, a stroke or trauma to the spinal cord, the circulatory system can collapse. Specialized treatment within a medical facility is required for neurogenic shock. There's nothing to do for it on your own except what you'd do for any type of shock: keep the victim warm, provide oxygen, give fluids if possible, and maintain an open airway.

5

WILD THINGS— BITES AND STINGS

POP QUIZ

The young woman sat on the exam table and looked up with a frown. It seemed she'd been sitting outside on her lunch break and enticed a squirrel to eat out of her hand. The squirrel bit her, and she was worried about rabies.

What's the one thing she should *not* have done?

A. Wash the wound thoroughly and immediately with soap and water.

B. Ask the local health department what animals are likely to have rabies in the area.

C. Think of the squirrel more like you would a pet than a wild animal.

D. Not worry too much; healthy squirrels usually don't transmit rabies to humans.

A. Incorrect. Washing the wound thoroughly is a must. A bacterial infection, not rabies, is the most common complication from any bite. Besides, washing it thoroughly, as you'll see on page 100, washes away a portion of all germs, including the ones that cause rabies.

B. Incorrect. Calling the local health department could save you a set of rabies vaccines or alert you that your risk is high enough that you need to get it.

C. Correct. I'll bet (I hope) you know this one. Make sure your kids know this also—about all wild animals. In fact, make sure they know that dogs and cats can be unfriendly, too.

D. Incorrect. Any animal can have rabies, but usually if the disease is present, the animal will be sick. (Raccoons are an exception.) Also, small animals, when sick, will usually be quickly eaten by bigger animals. In other words, they're unlikely to be around long enough to pose a danger.

PREVENTING THE MOST COMMON PROBLEM

After any bite, bacterial infection is a concern. Sure, we all worry about venom, along with rabies and other diseases. But skin and soft-tissue infections are by far the most common problems. So cleaning the bitten area with soap and water and keeping it clean are vitally important.

Of course, it would be nice not to have to deal with these bites in the first place. So thwart bugs with a DEET-type insect repellent or your favorite alternative, such as citronella oil, lemongrass oil, geranium oil, or neem oil. Apply insect repellent to your pet, too. Wear long sleeves, and consider high-top boots with pants tucked into them or taped to the outside for added protection against snakes and ticks. Watch where you're walking, and don't stick your hand into a place you can't see. If mosquitoes are a problem, consider installing screens on windows and doors and using a net for sleeping.

SNAKEBITES

There are two general types of poisonous snakes in the United States: pit vipers and coral snakes.

Pit vipers have a heat sensor, called a pit, located on each side of the head between the nostril and eye. Their heads are triangular, and their eyes have elliptical pupils, which look like slits. Common types of pit vipers include rattlesnakes, copperheads, and water moccasins (cottonmouths).

Coral snakes have round pupils and sport yellow, red, and black rings on their bodies. They can be confused with some types of nonpoisonous milk snakes—which use constriction to kill their prey—but although there are ways to tell the difference, there are exceptions, so stay away from all three.

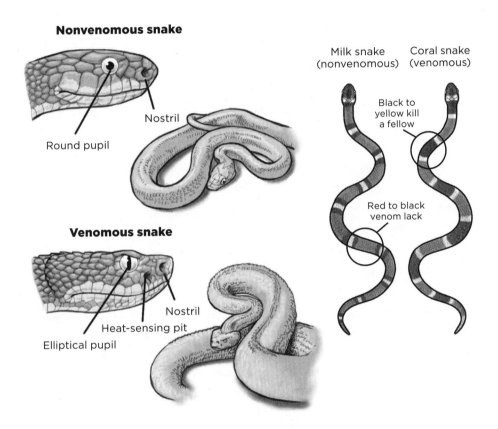

Nonvenomous snake

Round pupil

Nostril

Milk snake (nonvenomous) Coral snake (venomous)

Black to yellow kill a fellow

Red to black venom lack

Venomous snake

Elliptical pupil

Heat-sensing pit

Nostril

SIGNS YOU'VE BEEN BITTEN BY A VENOMOUS SNAKE

Nonvenomous snakebites tend to leave a row of several small puncture wounds from the animal's many teeth. But a bite from a venomous snake will also leave from one to four larger fang marks. (A new set of fangs could be coming in while the old set is still in place.) Venomous bites also usually bleed a lot more because the fangs penetrate more deeply into the flesh and because the venom itself can cause hemorrhaging.

Nonvenomous snake bite

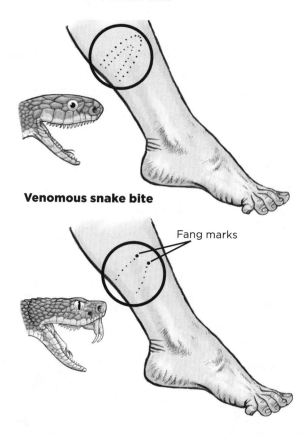

Venomous snake bite

Fang marks

If venom has been injected, the bitten area swells within ten to fifteen minutes. This is not always severe, but it can be—sometimes enough to cut off the circulation to the bitten extremity completely. If that happens, the flesh may need to be surgically and sterilely cut open to loosen the constriction.

Other clues you've been bitten by a venomous snake are:

• Severe pain, often a burning type, soon after the bite

• A metallic taste in your mouth or a numb tongue

• A tingling sensation or sweating

Hyperventilation from anxiety can also cause tingling and sweating. If you're unsure of the cause, slowing down your breathing or breathing into a bag for a minute or two will usually relieve the symptoms caused by anxiety, but not those caused by venom.

TREATMENT

If you get bitten—unless you really know your snakes and are sure the one that bit you is not venomous—seek expert help immediately. That's because the only thing that counteracts the effects of snake venom is antivenin.

That's not to say you'll always need antivenin. About 20 percent of bites from venomous snakes inject no venom. And only another 20 percent inject enough to be life-threatening. But you don't want to just wait around and see what happens, because if you do need the antivenin, getting it sooner rather than later can save your life.

While it helps to be able to identify the snake so that medical experts (if you can get to them) can determine whether you need antivenin, don't waste a lot of time trying to find it. And remember to remain wary of even dead snakes. They can strike from a distance of half the length of their bodies, and the strike reflex can remain for ninety minutes after they're dead—even if they've been decapitated. A good compromise would be to take a quick photo. But don't wade out into the tall grass searching.

Use your judgment to determine how much energy you should expend to get to expert help. Physical activity can speed up the spread of the venom through your system, but on the other hand you want to get the antivenin quickly if you need it.

If you need to travel over long distances, consider calling in air transfer if possible. Meantime you can try to slow down the spread of the venom by wrapping the area with an elastic bandage. (Though how much wrapping actually helps is still a matter of debate; some think that it keeps the venom more concentrated, making tissue damage more likely.) If you choose to try it, you'll need to wrap it tightly and cover the whole extremity. Check it regularly and loosen as needed if the circulation seems to be cutting off (that is, if you can detect no pulse in the wrist or foot).

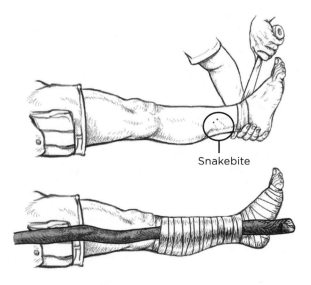

Snakebite

Immobilizing muscle movement may slow the spread of venom even further, so if the bite is on a leg, add a splint; if it's on an arm, put it in a sling. This may at least keep the muscles around the bite from pumping the venom into the rest of your body until you can get expert help and access to antivenin. Of course, that reasoning makes no sense if expert help is not going to be an option. So if you're on your own:

- Sit or lie down, depending on your symptoms. Feeling dizzy or faint can be a sign of low blood pressure. But shortness of breath could be caused by swelling in the lungs, which might be alleviated by sitting up. Bottom line: position yourself however you're most comfortable.

- Keep the bitten area level with your heart. Any lower could increase swelling. Any higher could increase the venom flow to the rest of your body.

- Take something for pain if you have it.

- Drink lots of fluids. In venomous bites a lot of fluid may be lost as a result of blood hemorrhaging into the tissues. In addition, cells and blood vessels in all parts of the body can start leaking, which can lead to severe dehydration. Consider an IV for fluids if it's available.

- Wash the wound, and keep the area clean.

You Could Be Allergic to Snakebites

Snake venom, just like bee, spider, ant, or any other venom, can cause a life-threatening allergic reaction called anaphylaxis. The symptoms, such as shortness of breath, hives, and feeling faint, occur within seconds or minutes after the bite, followed by severe difficulty breathing, shock, collapse, and heart stoppage. Whatever the cause, the treatment consists of getting a shot of epinephrine as soon as possible (such as from an EpiPen, a prescription device that many people who are severely allergic to something keep with them) and, of course, expert help if possible.

TREATMENT DON'TS

- Don't cut the wound or try to suck out the venom. There's no proof it helps, and it increases the risk the wound will get infected..

- Don't use a tourniquet. You'll endanger the tissue by cutting off circulation. In addition, completely concentrating the venom and then loosening the tourniquet ensures a quick burst of concentrated venom into the system that can cause more harm than if it were allowed to disperse on its own.

SPIDER BITES

In the United States, the brown recluse, the hobo, and the black widow are the three spiders that cause harm to humans. Often the culprit is never seen: the only evidence of a bite is the damage the venom causes. And it can be pretty specific; in most cases, the type of damage can tell you what kind of spider bit you.

Brown recluses like their privacy. They stay under seldom-used boxes, under sheets on the bed, or under anything that hasn't been disturbed for a few hours. The bite causes little or no initial pain. But within a few hours the area can really start throbbing.

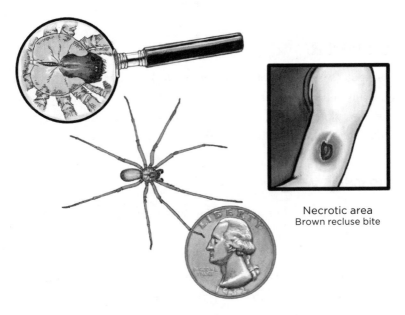

Necrotic area
Brown recluse bite

A brown recluse spider and its bite

Clues

Your first clue to a brown recluse bite can be a painful black dot where the venom is killing skin tissue. This could happen several minutes or a few hours after the bite. The damage may stay small and superficial, or the wound could become deep and wide, perhaps a couple of inches across. Victims occasionally have fever and feel ill.

Complications

As the dead skin sloughs off, if the damage is deep, the wound underneath can take weeks to heal. Like with any wound, infection is a risk. Some wounds are large enough to cause obvious scars—or even to need skin grafts to heal.

Treatment

Cool compresses or ice packs can help the pain. As always, keep a cloth between the skin and the ice pack, and only keep the pack on for ten minutes at a time to avoid skin damage from excessive cold. Pain medicine can also help, since the pain can be severe.

Clean the wound once or twice a day. Cover it if it's likely to get dirty, but don't try to remove the thick, black, dead skin, called an eschar. Letting it slough off on its own will cause less damage to the underlying healthy skin. Antibiotics may be needed if there are signs of infection (see page 16).

HOBO SPIDER

The hobo spider's bite is similar to the brown recluse's but usually causes less skin damage, if any. The spider can be difficult to identify, because its appearance varies. If you have skin damage and find the spider and it's not a brown recluse, the hobo is the likely culprit. Treatment is the same.

BLACK WIDOW

The black widow likes to live under places such as eaves, porches, and woodpiles.

Clues

Often a black widow's bite is felt as a little sting or pinprick, but sometimes there's no sensation at all. Usually, skin damage is minimal. Sometimes the only evidence of a bite is two tiny fang marks—if you can find them.

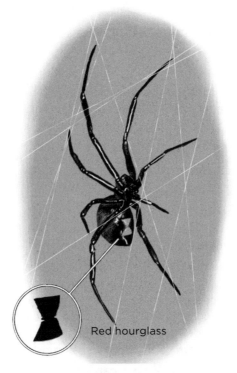

Red hourglass

The female black widow spider can be identified by the red hourglass shape on her belly.

After several minutes to a few hours, severe muscle pain and cramping in the abdomen, limbs, chest, or back becomes the main clue, but unless you suspect a bite, you may not recognize it's the cause of the symptoms. In fact, the pain can be confused with that of a heart attack, appendicitis, and other serious problems. If you have doubts, get an expert opinion whenever possible.

Your blood pressure may get very high. Nausea, vomiting, and sweating can occur. Seizures and even death are possible but rare. Severe symptoms are more common in small children and elderly people.

Treatment

Cool compresses around the bite site help with the pain, as do muscle relaxants, pain medicine, and warm soaks in the area of cramping. The pain usually goes away in a few days. Antivenin is occasionally given, more often in young children and elderly people.

Antivenin Pros and Cons

Whether you use the term "antivenom" or "antivenin," you're talking about a medicine chock-full of antibodies to a specific venom. It's like an injectable SWAT team that neutralizes venom. It can't do anything for the damage done. Rather, it prevents further damage. The sooner you give it, the less risk the venom will have time to cause organ damage. So why not give it to everyone who's been bitten by a spider or snake?

1. It can cause a sudden, life-threatening anaphylactic reaction or serum sickness—a fever and feeling ill for several weeks.

2. It can be hard to come by. That's been the case in Florida for coral-snake antivenin since 2013. The bite of a coral snake is so deadly that anyone bitten has been automatically given the antivenin. But it's getting harder to find enough snakes to be milked for their venom so the antivenin can be produced.

3. It's expensive. The cost can run into the tens of thousands of dollars.

   Of course, antivenin can also be lifesaving, so if you're bitten, your best bet is to get to a health care facility as soon as possible. You'll be monitored and only given the antivenin if you start showing early signs of internal damage.

MAMMAL BITES

In addition to injuring skin, an animal bite may tear and bruise muscle, blood vessels, nerves, and even bones. And it always introduces bacteria into these bitten areas. At minimum, irrigate the bite wound well and treat it like a puncture wound (see page 26).

In a health care facility, most animal bites aren't closed unless they're large and gaping or potentially disfiguring. Even then, it's a judgment call, since bites are very likely to become even more infected when closed.

In general, the larger the animal and the stronger the jaws, the greater the tissue damage and infection risk. But a couple of exceptions do come to mind. With any of these bites, seek expert care when it's available.

CAT BITES

Cats have needlelike teeth that can pierce deep into flesh without causing a lot of external damage. And their mouths usually contain a nasty bacterium called *Pasteurella multocida*, which can cause a quick and serious infection. The sooner antibiotics are started the better. Oral antibiotics that typically treat *Pasteurella* are amoxicillin-clavulanate (Augmentin), cefprozil (Cefzil), cefuroxime (Ceftin), and azithromycin (Zithromax).

BITES TO THE HAND

Your hands have a lot of shallow tendons and muscles. And relative to other parts of your body, they don't have the greatest blood supply for fighting off infection. So no matter the size of the animal, a bite to your hand is at high risk of serious infection.

Clean the bite vigorously, and start antibiotics if available. The ones mentioned in the previous section should treat both staph infections and infections from cat bites. As with any infection, these drugs may or may not work.

BITES FROM RABID ANIMALS

Rabies is rare in the United States, but it's deadly and has no cure. There is a vaccine, but you have to get it before symptoms begin. Certain animal handlers, cave explorers, and people traveling to countries with a high rabies risk may opt to get the vaccine series of three shots before exposure; the rest of us usually wait until after we've gotten a suspicious bite. Rabies symptoms usually start a month or more after exposure but can begin within a few days. If they do occur, you've waited too long.

If an animal bites you, contact the health department, animal control, or an animal shelter if you can to find out whether that type of animal is at risk for rabies in your area. If it is, you'll need rabies shots. If the animal can be captured, it may be penned up for ten days so it can be monitored for signs of rabies. (Don't try to capture the animal yourself. You'll only risk further exposure.)

Bat bites are always a worry. Depending on the region, raccoons, foxes, and skunks can be at high risk of having rabies. Even rabbits have been known to have it. Pet-wise, unvaccinated cats carry some of the highest risk but you should also beware of unvaccinated dogs and ferrets.

Treatment

Studies have shown that thorough wound cleaning can significantly decrease your risk of becoming infected with rabies. Pressure-irrigate (see page 22) the wound really well with one of the following, in order of preference:

- Povidone-iodine (Betadine)

- 2 percent benzalkonium chloride (Zephiran Chloride)

- Soap and water

- Plain water

These substances have been shown to get rid of much of the rabies bacteria and significantly decrease your risk of becoming infected.

If there's no expert help available, to dispose of a dead animal you suspect might have rabies, you'll need a mask, gloves, and a shovel to pick up the dead animal. If possible, add a waterproof apron along with goggles and a face mask. Spray the carcass thoroughly with a solution of at least one part chlorine to nine parts water, and bury the animal a foot or more below ground so other animals are less likely to dig it up. If you have some plastic, cover the animal before filling in the dirt.

> ### Why Bat Rabies is Sneaky
>
> Bats do a lot of good. They eat tons of insects. But some also have rabies. And people have been known to get rabies from contact with bats even when there was no known bite or scratch. The thinking is that their small, needlelike teeth can puncture the skin so finely that you may not be able to find a wound.
>
> So if you've had even possible contact with bats—say, you've been hit by a flying bat or discover you've been sleeping in a room with a bat—you should have rabies shots. People have been known to get rabies under both these circumstances without ever finding a wound.

BEE, WASP, AND FIRE ANT STINGS

Bees, wasps, and fire ants all inject venom that can cause life-threatening allergic reactions—whether you've been allergic before or not. A bee may leave its barbed stinger and venom sac stuck in your skin, still pumping venom. Brush it off as quickly as possible. Wasps don't have barbs, so they sting and fly away, keeping their stingers with them.

Here are some treatments that may help with the pain and itching from any of these stings:

- An ice pack (with a cloth placed between the skin and the pack), a cold, wet rag, or anything cold (such as a soda can or a bag of frozen vegetables) applied for no more than ten minutes at a time
- A paste of baking soda and water
- A cloth soaked in vinegar
- A paste of baking soda and vinegar
- A paste of meat tenderizer and water
- Wet tobacco

Oral medications usually aren't needed unless the local reaction is quite red and itchy or there are multiple stings, swelling, a rash, or a past history of allergic reactions. In such cases, an antihistamine such as diphenhydramine (Benadryl), or one of the "nondrowsy" ones, can be taken on a regular basis for a few days. A prescription steroid, such as prednisone, could be taken in the same way.

Keep the stung area clean to avoid infection. Many fire ant stings leave little pus-filled bumps. It's best to leave them alone and just keep them clean.

ANAPHYLAXIS

Anaphylaxis is a life-threatening allergic reaction that can occur after an insect sting, a spider bite, a snake bite, and many other venomous attacks. It can also occur after exposure to a medicine or food. In fact, just about anything can cause a severe allergic reaction in someone.

CLUES

These symptoms may start within a minute or up to two hours after exposure:

- Hives or welts anywhere on your body
- Swelling of your face, tongue, or throat
- Trouble breathing

- Fainting caused by a drop in blood pressure

- A tingling or funny taste in your mouth

TREATMENT

People with anaphylaxis need treatment right away.

- Immediately call 911 if possible.

- Use an EpiPen, a prescription device that injects epinephrine. Nothing works as well as epinephrine to treat an anaphylactic reaction. Anaphylaxis is possible even if you've never had a reaction, so check with your doctor about keeping an EpiPen on hand for emergencies.

- Lie down. Anaphylaxis makes your blood pressure fall, and lying down will help keep the blood flow going to your head and heart.

- An antihistamine, such as diphenhydramine (Benadryl), may or may not help, but it is worth a try if expert care is not immediately available. A prescription steroid is another alternative. Use both if available.

- An albuterol inhaler, commonly used for asthma, is worth a try if you have trouble breathing.

If you've had an allergic reaction from a sting or bite before, you should see an allergist for testing to see whether a series of shots can make you less allergic and decrease the severity of your next reaction. Think of it as a prep thing. Don't delay.

6

FACE FACTS

POP QUIZ

As I was finishing treatment of a four-year-old's cut, his mother piped up: "Oh, by the way, he's been saying 'Huh?' a lot lately. I've attributed it to habit, but since we're here, would you take a look in his ears?"

"No problem."

I wasn't really surprised to see something green peeking out of the canal in one ear—it was pushed just far enough in to not be obvious. It's what was in the other ear that surprised me.

Exactly the same thing.

Fortunately, the objects were shallow enough for me to pluck them out easily with my handy-dandy needle-nose tweezers. They turned out to be green peas. And, voilà, the boy could hear.

Out of the four options below, what should I *not* have done after that?

A. Look in the ear canals again, and if they weren't clear, consider irrigating them with some warm water from a syringe.

B. Call social services to report child neglect.

C. Check his hearing at a later date.

D. Consider some antibiotic drops.

ANSWERS

A. Incorrect. I'm a big proponent of irrigation. In fact, unless an object is close enough to the surface for me to grab hold of it easily, I go straight to irrigation. I've found it so much easier—and less traumatic.

B. Correct. There are many reasons to call social services, but finding a foreign body in the ear is not one of them. Over my years of treating kids, I've decided that for many children, sticking something in their ears or nostrils, at least once, seems a rite of passage. Crayons, toy cars, toy soldiers, food, beads, rocks—whatever will fit, I've found it.

C. Incorrect. In a few days, after the excitement has died down, I'd think it a good idea to have this boy's hearing checked—without the peas—just to make sure nothing else is going on. In fact, it's a good idea for all children periodically.

D. Incorrect. Because any irritation of the canals could increase the risk of infection, a few drops of antibiotics in the ears for a few days is a good precaution. Of course if the canals look raw and red, this is a must. A mixture of vinegar and water is an alternative if you can't get the antibiotics.

EYES

I'm often amazed at the fact that the tiniest scratch of the cornea or speck of debris in the eye can cause enough discomfort to disrupt a person's life. But unless it goes really deep, a scratch that causes such ultrasensitivity can quickly heal without any scarring or residual damage. On the other hand, damage that penetrates the deeper layers of the eye can be irreversible.

So to avoid annoyance—and worse—protect your eyes. Wear goggles for clearing brush and for metal or carpentry work. Even if you wear glasses, get protective side shields for such tasks.

In the sun, no matter the season, wear sunglasses that guarantee 99 to 100 percent UVA (ultraviolet A) and UVB (ultraviolet B) protection.

FOREIGN BODIES

Mama was right. If you feel something in your eye, don't rub it. You may cause whatever's in there to scratch your cornea, and then you've got a second problem.

(The cornea is the clear covering over the colored part of the eye and the pupil, and it's very sensitive. The covering over the white part is a lot less so.)

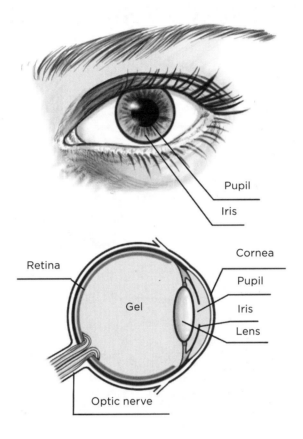

Diagnosis

If it feels like something is in your eye, look in a mirror or get someone to check your eye. You may see a speck, sometimes very tiny. Shining a flashlight on your eye, first directly, then at an angle, can help you see it. A magnifying glass may also help. If you see nothing, flip your lid (see page 106).

Treatment for Simple Specks

If you're wearing contact lenses, take out the one in your affected eye.

If you see the object, you can try dabbing it out with a damp cloth or cotton swab. Otherwise, try flushing it out with clean water. If you still feel something, flush again. If that doesn't work, you may have a scratched cornea.

✚ HOW TO FLIP YOUR LID AND FIND A SPECK THAT'S HIDING

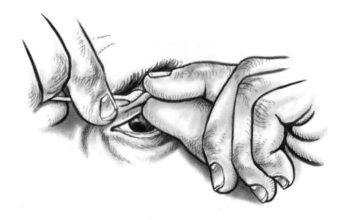

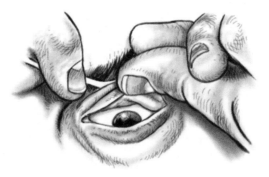

If you think something's in your eye but can't find it, here's a trick. Wash your hands, and get two cotton swabs. Dampen one of them with water.

1. Place the dry swab over the upper eyelid.

2. While looking downward, grab the edge of the lid with your thumb and index finger. Because you're looking down, you should be touching the less sensitive, white part of the eye. Be careful not to scratch your eye with your fingernail.

3. Quickly flip the lid up, inside out, and over the swab. Look for debris.

4. Let go of the dry swab, and remove any debris with the dampened swab.

Treatment for Embedded Specks

Sometimes debris can become embedded in the cornea; if it does, it's impossible to dab or wash out.

Occasionally, a magnet will pull out a metal speck. Make sure the magnet is very clean, and just barely touch the speck when you try to get it out.

If this doesn't work, the speck may need to be removed by a medical professional using something like a sterile needle. Don't try this on your own. Not only is it virtually impossible to do without some anesthetic, you're also likely to do more harm than good.

Until you can get help, for symptom relief, consider patching your eye to keep it tightly closed. Otherwise every blink will cause irritation when the lid touches the object. Even with the patch, consider sunglasses if you must go outside, because if one eye is exposed to bright light, both pupils will react, and this may cause discomfort in the patched eye. Remember that you need both eyes working for proper depth perception. So avoid driving or doing anything else that requires knowing how close or far away something is.

SCRATCHED CORNEA

When you have a scratched cornea, it feels just like something is in your eye. Sometimes the fact that you have a scratch is obvious—say, if you know that a tree branch or your fingernail rubbed against your eye. Other times, you may not know anything touched your eye: a small foreign body you didn't see might have scratched it, for example.

Diagnosis

I've had dozens of patients tell me they know for a fact that something's in their eye because of the way it feels. It's hard to convince them otherwise—until I get them to look in the mirror. One drop of fluorescein, or a little touch to the corner of the eye with a fluorescein strip, spreads a dye that highlights even the tiniest scratch in a green or yellow hue. A black light makes it really stand out, but most dyed scratches can be seen without one.

Of course, you probably won't have any fluorescein, which isn't sold over the counter. But often you can see the scratch without it. It helps to place a flashlight close to the outside corner of your eye and shine it crosswise toward your nose. If that doesn't work, you may have to go on the assumption that since it feels like something's in your eye and you've looked for it thoroughly and can't find it, it's likely a scratch.

Treatment

Unless the scratch has punctured all the way through the cornea (see below), it will typically heal within twenty-four to forty-eight hours. Some scratches can take longer to heal, even up to a week, and it's hard to predict which ones will. Depending on your comfort level, you can patch the eye shut—or not. Either way, it should heal. If you have prescription antibiotic eyedrops, use them to prevent the scratch from getting infected.

CORNEAL ULCER

A corneal ulcer feels like a scratch, but most corneal ulcers are caused by a virus. Fluorescein will reveal a pinhole-size spot of erosion. Sometimes you can see it with a flashlight.

Without expert help, a corneal ulcer should be treated the same way a scratch would be. But it's especially important to use antibiotic eyedrops if you have any, because some corneal ulcers are caused by bacteria and could be cured with the drops. Most corneal ulcers are from a virus infection and will heal in a few days, but others can get worse, even damaging the eye permanently. Unfortunately, unless you can get expert care, there's nothing else you can do.

PENETRATING EYE WOUND

If you think something may have punctured the eye beyond the outside layers, one of the dangers is that some of the eye's gel-like substance, or vitreous fluid, may leak out. This can cause everything else inside the globe of the eye to shift, resulting in significant loss of vision. In case of a penetrating wound:

- Don't apply any pressure to the eye.
- Don't remove the object unless there's no way you can get help for several days. Removing the object will likely cause further damage. But if you decide you have to remove it, continue to protect the eye from pressure.
- Until you can get expert help, consider making an eyecup to protect against accidental bumping. For example, cut the bottom out of a paper cup and tape it to the bony area around the eye.

PINKEYE

The cause of pinkeye is usually a very contagious virus. So if you're around other people and no one else has it or gets it, the cause of your misery is likely allergies or something other than pinkeye.

If you have pinkeye, your eye may swell a bit and ooze a kind of pus. About half the time, it will eventually infect the other eye.

Alternatives to Antibiotic Eyedrops

Studies regarding the effectiveness and side effects of alternatives to antibiotic eyedrops are scarce. If you have no prescription antibiotic eyedrops, and you're not going to be able to get expert help for several days, you'll have to decide whether using an alternative is worth the risk of making the problem worse, especially since many eye infections are viral, and the drops won't help those. On the other hand, bacterial infections of the eye can be devastating. Below is a list of things you can try:

- **Antibacterial ointment made up of the same ingredients as the eyedrops (neomycin, gentamicin, or bacitracin):** The downside here is that there's no guarantee that the ointment is completely sterile, and it might contain preservatives that could cause irritation.

- **Raw honey:** This has been proved to kill bacteria in skin wounds (see page 26). About a tablespoon of it mixed with a cup of clean water makes a good flush. Make sure the honey is not grainy, which could scratch the eye. There's a risk of dangerous botulism infection in kids less than two years old.

- **Colloidal silver drops:** Found at health-food and nutritional-supplement stores, colloidal silver drops are controversial. Many people swear by them, but multiple studies have shown that they're ineffective—and, if enough is swallowed over a period of time, potentially dangerous. For eye infections, since you put the drops in your eye rather than ingest them, the most likely harm is probably irritation.

Whichever of these alternative remedies you choose, use it every four to six hours for seven days, or until two days after the symptoms are gone, whichever span of time is longer. If the infection hasn't gone away after about two weeks, stop. The remedy is likely to not be working, and continuing it increases the risk that side effects will develop.

Treatment

Throw away any contact lenses you were using near or at the onset of symptoms. Don't use new ones until all the symptoms have been gone for a couple of days.

Holding a warm, wet cloth to your eye can be quite soothing. If the cause is viral, pinkeye will run its course in a few days. But sometimes the cause is bacterial. It's even hard for doctors to tell the difference. So if you have prescription antibiotic eye drops, consider using them.

Prevention

If someone close to you has pinkeye, you're probably next. Wash your hands with soap and water often. Use disinfectant cleaners on surfaces such as doorknobs and tools. Throw away eye makeup that could be contaminated. Don't use the same bottle of eyedrops the infected person is using.

STY

A sty is a clogged-up, sometimes infected oil gland—think pimple—on the eyelid. Many sties go away without treatment. But it's hard to predict which will go away and which will get worse, so it's usually worth your while to treat them.

Apply heat to your eyelid. Moist heat is better—for example, a cloth dampened with warm water (not hot enough to burn). Apply it over and over again—maybe at least ten minutes every two hours. Some people apply warm, moist tea bags or something else that might hold warmth a little longer than a cloth.

Even if the whole eyelid is swollen and red, the sty should shrink down to smaller than the size of a pea within a day or two. From there, it may drain out a little pus or just go away.

If the heat isn't working after a day and getting to a doctor is impossible, you can try prescription antibiotic eye ointment if you have it. If the infection is getting worse, take oral antibiotics if you have them, and try extra hard to get to that doctor.

Never squeeze a sty, and never poke a sty with a needle. Doing either is likely to spread the infection and make it much worse.

> ### DOCTOR SPEAK
>
> A chalazion is an eyelid cyst or an area of scar tissue that sometimes forms after a sty has healed. Leave it alone. When you can see a doctor you can have it surgically removed if you wish. Other than being a nuisance, it shouldn't cause trouble unless it gets reinfected. Then you'd simply treat it like a sty.

✚ HOW TO MAKE YOUR OWN PINHOLE GLASSES

If you're nearsighted and break your glasses in a survival situation, you can use this trick to create makeshift glasses. The technique is based on the age-old knowledge that looking through a pinhole makes you see more clearly—same as squinting, only better. The pinhole limits scattered light and focuses what's left directly onto the retina (the back of the eye, which sends visual signals to the brain).

1. Start with any opaque material—paper, cardboard, duct tape with the sticky sides stuck together—the thinner the better, as long as light can't get through.

2. Punch a few pinholes of various small sizes into it using something like a safety pin or paper clip. Look through the different sizes to see which works best.

3. Looking through a pinhole greatly limits your field of vision, so combat that by punching a bunch more pinholes of the size you've decided best.

4. Attach these makeshift lenses to a glasses frame. Or make your own frame from sticks or cardboard, or tape the lenses to a headband made of cloth—anything to get you by.

   Try to wear sunglasses with these pinhole glasses if you're outside.

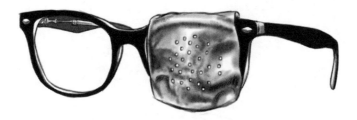

Despite rumors to the contrary, pinhole glasses will not correct your vision in any permanent manner. This is a temporary fix, and I doubt it will become a fashion statement. But it solves a common fear that many of us blurry-eyed sorts have about surviving disasters.

BOTTOM LINE ON MANAGEMENT OF EYE PROBLEMS

There are far too many things that can go wrong with the eyes to mention them all here. Many conditions need a specialized exam and care. Here are a few general concepts to keep in mind if professional help is impossible to get:

- If the flesh around the eye is red or painful, apply heat, and start antibiotic drops if you have them. If the redness, tenderness, or swelling involves the skin beyond the eyelid, change to oral antibiotics if you have them. Some of these infections can become serious and even cause blindness.

- If you have pain in the eye or vision loss resulting from anything other than an infection or a scratch, it's potentially serious, but there's not much you can do until you get expert help.

- Unless you have a puncture wound, you can't go wrong with clean-water flushing (as long as you take your contact lenses out first). Flush at least fifteen minutes—more like thirty if you think a bad irritant has gotten in your eye—or until the symptoms subside.

EARS

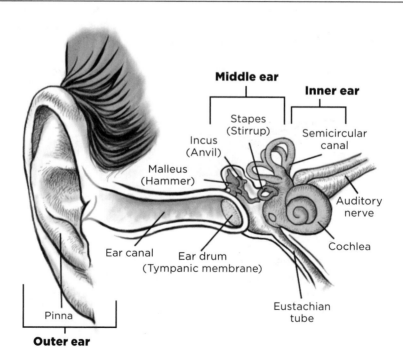

In general, we can divide ear problems into three categories:

- **The outer, or external, ear i**ncludes the parts you can see, along with the ear canal. It ends with the eardrum.

- **The middle ear** is located just behind the eardrum. It consists of three small bones. When the eardrum vibrates with sound, those bones carry the vibrations to the inner ear. The eustachian tube drains fluid from the middle and inner ear to the back of the nose near the throat, where you swallow it. Except for this single opening, the middle and inner ear are completely enclosed, unless there's a leak in the eardrum. In addition to draining fluid, the tube keeps air pressure in the middle and inner ear equal to the outside pressure. If the tube stops up because of inflammation, swelling, or infection anywhere along its course, air pressure, fluid, or both can build up, causing possible hearing loss and discomfort. If there's too much fluid or pressure, the eardrum will spring a leak to release it. Sometimes the leak causes pain, but often, by relieving the pressure, it does just the opposite. Either way, if the eustachian tube starts draining again, the leak usually heals with time.

- **The inner ear** has two parts. The cochlea turns the vibrations into impulses that the brain deciphers as sound. The semicircular canal controls balance and equilibrium. The auditory nerve connects the inner ear directly to your brain. Any damage in the area from the eardrum to the nerve will impair hearing.

OUTER EAR

The two most common external-ear problems are infection and ear canal blockage. These things can happen separately or together.

Infection

Irritation of the canal by something like a cotton swab, a hairpin, or earplugs can give bacteria an entry into the skin, where they can set up shop. Also, chronically wet ear canals not only damage the skin but also allow certain bacteria to thrive. (You've heard of swimmer's ear?)

Clues that someone may have an external-ear infection are:

- **Pain:** It hurts to wiggle or press on the external part of the ear.

- **Redness:** If you look in the canal with an otoscope (that thing that health care providers use to examine your ear), it's red and may be swollen.

It's important to start prescription antibiotic eardrops early, because the longer you wait, the more swollen the canal can get. In fact, it can get so swollen that the drops can't make it all the way down. In those cases a doctor may insert something called an earwick into the ear. That's a small, sticklike device made of wicking material that can be pushed into a swollen canal. The end of the earwick is left protruding slightly so it can be removed after the swelling goes down. With the earwick in, when you administer eardrops, the material draws the medicine into the ear. Inserting the earwick hurts like the dickens, though. Never try this technique unless you have an earwick and know what you're doing because otherwise you're likely to damage the ear..

If you don't have antibiotic eardrops, oral antibiotics work, but they take longer. If you have a mild infection or don't have antibiotics, you can try using a few drops of white vinegar mixed with a couple of drops of rubbing alcohol. Caution: the alcohol may sting. Use the drops every four hours while awake for a week.

To try to prevent an ear canal infection, first, never clean your ear with anything smaller than your finger. In most people, the little hairs along the canal, aided by the movement of your jaw while you chew your food (which in turn makes the ear canal move), gradually usher the wax out. Cotton swabs irritate the canal and can even pack the wax in so far that the hairs can't help it get out. Earplugs can do the same.

Also, watch the water immersion. Water turns earwax into mush, which, if left in place, exposes the ear to constant moisture. If you think there's a little water in your ear, you can help dry it out with a couple of drops of rubbing alcohol. A hair dryer set on low heat can work, but don't risk a burn by using it for too long or by holding it too close to the ear. If it's loud, it may not be great for your hearing, either.

Blockage

There are two main things that cause blockage in the ears:

- **Earwax:** Some people just produce too much, but the vast majority of wax blockages are caused by packing it in with the infamous cotton swabs, earplugs, or ear buds.
- **Foreign objects:** This could be anything from a bug to a piece of cotton. In children, it could be virtually anything they can stuff in.

The big clue that there's blockage is a simple one: unexplained muffled hearing in one ear. If you have an otoscope, you can see the wax, if that's the problem. If the culprit is a foreign object, sometimes you can see it without a scope.

For earwax buildup, if you have some commercial earwax softening drops (sold over the counter), you can use those for a few nights before bedtime. With this method, often the wax comes out on its own while you sleep. You may or may not see it, but you'll know it's out because you're hearing better. Even if the drops don't work, they'll make the wax easier to irrigate out (see below). Other drops that seem to help include Colace liquid stool softener or household-strength hydrogen peroxide.

By the way, if you have ongoing trouble with wax buildup, putting the drops in once or twice a week can help keep it soft enough for the ear hairs and the movement from chewing food to do their job.

For a foreign body in the ear, if you see it, you can try to pluck it out with tweezers, but be careful not to just push it in farther in. Another way to get the thing out is to put a tiny bit of glue on a cotton swab, touch the object, wait a couple of minutes, and pull. Of course the obvious potential problem is that you might get glue in the ear.

For a live bug, put a few drops of alcohol in the ear to kill it, then irrigate it out.

✚ HOW TO IRRIGATE YOUR EAR CANAL

Irrigation is a great way to remove any foreign body or wax buildup in the ear.

1. Pour clean, lukewarm water into a bowl. (Using water that's too hot or cold can stimulate the auditory nerve—which also controls your balance—and cause dizziness.) Add a few drops of household-strength hydrogen peroxide if you wish.

2. Hold a towel or another bowl under the affected ear to catch the water as it comes out.

3. Using the water in the bowl, fill up a bulb syringe, a medical syringe without the needle, or a plastic bag or bottle with a pinhole in the bottom.

4. With the arm that's opposite the ear (for example, your left arm if you're irrigating your right ear), reach around the back of your head, grab your ear, and pull back and slightly upward.

5. Squeeze the bag, bulb, or whatever you're using so the water squirts into the ear canal with steady pressure.

6. You're finished when the object or glob of wax comes out. Stop if the irrigation hasn't worked within about five minutes or if you have pain or dizziness. You can try again in a few hours. By that time the wax, if that's your problem, should be even softer.

7. After you're done, put a couple of drops of alcohol (mixed with peroxide if you want) in your ear to help dry up excess water.

Perforated Eardrum

One patient I saw with a perforated eardrum had been waterskiing and fell on his side. He heard a hiss, felt pain, and noticed a dramatic drop in his hearing. He also got very dizzy. With time the hole healed on its own, and his hearing went back to normal.

Another of my patients wasn't so lucky. He was standing in the bathroom cleaning his ear with a cotton swab. His wife opened the door, which hit his elbow, and he poked the cotton swab through his eardrum. Talk about painful. He had a surgical repair and still has hearing loss.

A perforated eardrum can be caused by:

- A sudden burst of air pressure hitting the eardrum, as in the waterskiing case. A slap on the ear could do the same thing.

- Direct trauma, as in the cotton swab case.

- Pressure from the inside. If the eustachian tube isn't working correctly, fluid can build up to the point where the pressure causes a leak. Or a sudden, drastic change of barometric pressure, like what happens when you fly, could do the damage.

You might suspect a perforated eardrum if any of the following happens:

- There's trauma or pressure to the ear followed by immediately hearing loss, sometimes with a hissing sound.

- Severe pain from a middle ear infection is suddenly relieved (when the leak relieves the pressure buildup).

- Cloudy fluid—pus—starts leaking out of the ear canal.

If you have an otoscope, you might be able to see the hole. But until you can get expert help, just leave a perforated eardrum alone. Many small holes heal on their own. Keep liquid out of the ear. Avoid quick movements of the head, which might trigger dizziness. And stay away from heights and dangerous machines, because you could suddenly lose your balance without warning.

MIDDLE EAR

When things go wrong in the middle ear, you can get temporary hearing loss, an ear infection, or even a bone infection.

Fluid Buildup: Otitis Media with Effusion

Otitis media with effusion, also called serous otitis—let's just call it OME—is simply a buildup of fluid in the middle ear without infection. Normally, the tissues in the middle ear secrete a little fluid, which drains out the eustachian tube. If the tube gets stopped up or swollen—from a cold, nasal allergies, or reasons unknown—the fluid builds up. This can result in a decrease in hearing that's virtually indistinguishable from the hearing loss brought on by impacted wax or a foreign body.

Two clues that hearing loss might be caused by OME could be:

• You have nasal stuffiness, which could also affect the eustachian tube.

• Your ear canal is clear, confirmed with an otoscope check.

OME can also cause subtle changes in the eardrum, but these are difficult to detect unless you've looked in a lot of ears. Sometimes there's dizziness.

Usually, with time, the swelling or whatever is stopping up the eustachian tube will go away, and the fluid will start draining normally again down the back of the throat. You can try to hurry it along by taking a decongestant for a few days, using a humidifier, and gargling with warm water every few hours, but most often the problem will resolve in its own sweet time.

Occasionally the eustachian tube can stay stopped up for months no matter what you do. In that case, if it's driving you crazy, lancing of the eardrum by an ear, nose, and throat surgeon is an option. In fact, draining by lancing—and the insertion of tubes to continue to the drainage—is done a little sooner in children than in adults to reverse the potential for hearing loss, which could impair learning. Adults? Hey, we've already learned enough.

Infection: Acute Otitis Media

When most people think of an ear infection, especially in children, they're usually thinking of acute otitis media. AOM happens when viruses or bacteria get in through the eustachian tube and can't drain out because the tube isn't working well. With time and enough germ accumulation, the problem can grow into a full-blown infection. Since children's and adult's ears are different—for one thing, the eustachian tube is shorter in kids—children are more vulnerable to AOM.

In addition to pain inside the ear, acute otitis media may cause hearing loss, dizziness, and fever. The eardrum, seen through an otoscope, is red or grayish. Lymph nodes on the side of the neck under the infected ear can be tender and swollen. Sometimes the infection is preceded by a cold or another type of upper respiratory infection.

There's no great way to know if the infection is viral or bacterial, but if you're one of the 60 percent of infected people who start getting better in twenty-four hours without antibiotics, it's probably viral and will go away on its own.

If you do start antibiotics, take them for the fully recommended time. Amoxicillin is often effective, but some ear infections are resistant to it. Virtually any other oral antibiotic will usually do the job.

If the ear feels stopped up, the same treatments as for fluid buildup may help. For pain, you can try an over-the-counter pain reliever or prescription numbing drops if you have them.

Placing something warm over the ear may help with the pain, too, as can putting a few drops of warm oil in the ear. Some people find that garlic oil or mullein oil works. Just make sure the drops aren't too hot.

Complications of Ear Infections

Ear infections can lead to meningitis (a spinal cord infection), mastoiditis (an infection of a bone behind the ear), and other bone infections. Although these are fairly uncommon, they can be life-threatening, and the sooner the victim gets expert help the better.

One clue that suggests meningitis is a painful and stiff neck. A baby will become very irritable and difficult to comfort. An infection of the bone will cause tenderness to the bone in the area of infection. The bottom line is that someone with an ear infection who looks pretty sick should be checked out as soon as possible.

INNER EAR

As a young child, I thought it was fun to spin around until I couldn't stand. Now it just makes me sick to my stomach. But spinning is a great way to experience the usual symptoms of inner ear problems—loss of balance and nausea. Your eyes also flick furiously back and forth, trying to get in sync with what your inner ear is experiencing.

Causes of true inner ear problems include infections of the inner or middle ear, tumors, fluid, and anything that causes inflammation in that area. Symptoms range from a slight queasiness or unsteady sensation to a feeling that you or the room is spinning (vertigo). The feeling may be constant or come in waves.

If the underlying problem can be found, it should be treated. For nausea relief, any of the following may help:

- **An oral medication:** Prescription options include promethazine, ondansetron, and meclizine. Lower-strength meclizine is also available over the counter

(Dramamine Less Drowsy is one brand name). Learn any medication's side effects, interactions, and complications before taking it.

- **A little ginger:** If you drink ginger ale, make sure it contains actual ginger.

- **Acupressure:** Press your thumb to the middle of your opposite inner forearm, about two inches from the base of your palm. It may take thirty seconds to a few minutes for the nausea to subside.

- **Pressure-point motion sickness bracelets:** These are often available at pharmacies.

Also get some rest; avoid quick movements and driving; and avoid spicy foods, caffeine, and alcohol. Since the symptoms can come and go, stay away from situations in which losing your balance could result in injury.

Benign Paroxysmal Positional Vertigo (or Why the Room Won't Stop Spinning)

BPPV is a pretty common cause of inner ear problems, and it has a specific treatment that often works as a cure.

Inside your inner ear, calcium crystals reside in a gel-like substance. They can get dislodged due to head trauma, advancing age, or some unknown trigger. If enough crystals get loose, they can sometimes form a tiny stone or stones that move around and irritate the ear's delicate balance sensors. That causes benign paroxysmal positional vertigo. With BPPV, the feeling of spinning (vertigo) can be intense, but it comes and goes (that's why it's called paroxysmal) and is brought on by moving your head into certain positions, especially when you're lying down (which is why it's called positional).

So you might suspect BPPV if the room seems to be moving or spinning only when you're looking up or lying in certain positions. The symptoms usually last only a few seconds and not more than a couple of minutes.

A test called the Dix-Hallpike maneuver can aid in diagnosing BPPV. To make sure it's done properly and the results interpreted correctly, the test should be performed by an experienced health care provider. At a minimum, it helps if another person is there to hold your head and examine your eyes. Certainly never try it without a health care provider if you have known neck problems, because the maneuver could make the problems worse.

DIX-HALLPIKE MANEUVER

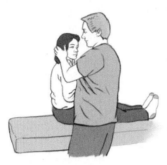

1. *Sit on a bed or table in a position such that when you lie back, your head will hang off the end. (Or you could just put a pillow under your neck.)*

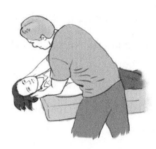

2. *Have someone turn your head forty-five degrees to the right, and keep your eyes open during the entire procedure.*

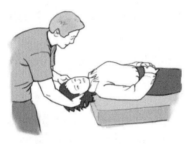

3. *While your partner holds your turned head, lie back until your head hangs off the back of the table toward the floor at a thirty-degree angle—eyes still open, the head still turned forty-five degrees to the right.*

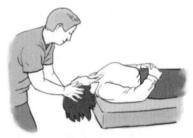

4. *Have your partner check your eyes: the test is positive if lying back brings on symptoms or if your partner sees your eyes rapidly darting to one side or the other (a condition called nystagmus).*

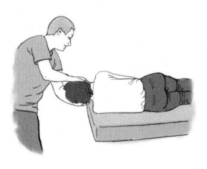

5. *If the test is negative, lie in a comfortable position for a few minutes to make sure you have no increased dizziness.*

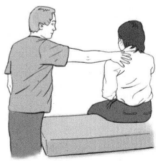

6. *Slowly sit back up, and repeat the test with your head turned to the left.*

EPLEY MANEUVER

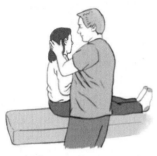

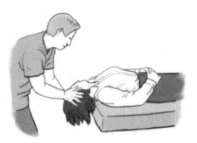

1. *Start in the same sitting position as you did for the Dix-Hallpike maneuver—with a partner holding your turned head forty-five degrees in the direction that brings on the symptoms.*

2. *With your partner holding your head, lie back until your head is hanging off the table, bed, or pillow and angled about thirty degrees toward the floor (again, just like in the previous maneuver). Hold that position for thirty seconds or until the vertigo symptoms subside, whichever comes first.*

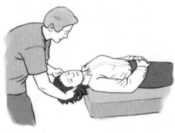

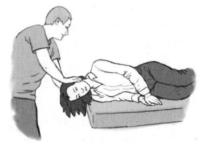

3. *Turn your head in the opposite direction and position it forty-five degrees from center. Wait the allotted time, as in step 2.*

4. *While your head is still in that position, roll on your side so your face is somewhat toward the floor. Wait the allotted time.*

5. *With your head still in that position and your body on its side, sit back up. Again wait the allotted time.*

6. *Repeat steps 1 through 5 until symptoms have subsided, but do not repeat the maneuver more than three times.*

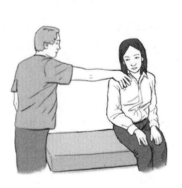

7. *Sit still in a comfortable position for twenty minutes. Then slowly stand.*

If the test confirms you have BPPV, the Epley maneuver may fix it.

At least the first try at the Epley maneuver should be done in a medical office, if possible, to make sure it's done properly and that it helps the symptoms: if it doesn't, perhaps there's another cause for the vertigo. And, as with the Dix-Hallpike maneuver, tell your provider if you have any neck problems.

Try to avoid bending your head up or down for the rest of the day. For five nights, avoid sleeping in the position that originally caused symptoms. Perform this maneuver at least once a day for a week or at least until you've been symptom-free for twenty-four hours.

About half the time this is a permanent cure. But if the symptoms come back, repeat the whole sequence.

NOSE

That big snout of yours is not just for looks. It filters and humidifies incoming air. And to warm that air, the nostrils contain a lot of blood vessels close to the surface. If the surface gets dry or broken, there can be a whole lot of bleeding.

I've treated quite a few nosebleeds, and, as with bleeds in other areas, applying direct pressure will usually stop one. The mistake many people make is thinking that holding their head back and putting an ice bag on their nose will stop the bleeding. The only thing tilting the head back does is allow the blood to run down the back of your throat and choke you. And the ice bag? Well, it can help slow the bleeding by constricting blood vessels, but it won't shut them down. The key is not ice or the position of your nose. It's direct pressure.

HOW TO STOP A NOSEBLEED

When your nose is bleeding, sitting is preferable to lying down. This lowers the blood pressure in the nose, making it easier to stop the bleeding. But if you feel dizzy, don't risk fainting. Lie down or put your head between your knees, and just apply a bit more pressure.

Unless you're lying down, tilt your head forward to allow the blood to drain out instead of down your throat. This is especially important in children or others who might be prone to suck the blood down their windpipes.

To stop the bleeding:

1. Pinch together the fleshy part of the nose next to (just below) the bony part. This alone stops most bleeding by applying direct pressure to the most likely source. Keep it pinched for about ten minutes.

2. If the bleeding hasn't stopped completely after ten minutes, pinch one nostril closed, then the other, to determine which side the bleeding is coming from.

3. Pack the bleeding side with a tampon, cotton balls, gauze, or other clean cloths. Stuff them in tightly to apply pressure. It may be a little uncomfortable. Coating the material first with a lubricant, such as K-Y Jelly, petroleum jelly, or an antibacterial ointment, can make this easier. Consider spraying the packing with a small amount of blood-vessel constrictor, such as Afrin or Neo-Synephrine, before you put it in. Don't do this if you have high blood pressure, though, even if your blood pressure is being treated and under control. If there's still bleeding, but it stops when you pinch the nostrils, you likely need more packing.

4. Place a piece of tape over the nostril to keep the packing in place for twenty-four to forty-eight hours. Before removing the packing, tilting your head back and applying a few drops of water to soak the packing material can keep it from sticking to the nasal lining.

POSTERIOR NOSEBLEED (WAY BACK THERE)

If bleeding doesn't stop with pinching or packing, it's possible you have what's called a posterior nosebleed, which is too far back for the packing to help. About 5 percent of nosebleeds fall into this category. Since posterior nosebleeds tend to involve an artery, you can lose a lot of blood fast. Getting expert medical help quickly can save your life.

If medical help is unavailable, you can try to pack the posterior nosebleed yourself, but the process is tricky and potentially more hazardous than anterior packing. Too much pressure could cause its own damage by cutting off circulation. Even worse, if something gets unattached that's been placed in the posterior part of the nose or throat, it could be inhaled down the windpipe. Of course, losing blood from a major nosebleed is dangerous, too. Needless to say, getting expert help is by far the safest route.

There are commercially available double-balloon catheters made just for this purpose. If you have one, that's your best bet. It should come with instructions. A similar option is a Foley catheter (for more on what a Foley is, see page 213).

FOREIGN BODY

If you have a foreign body stuck in the nose, you can try grabbing it with tweezers or forceps if you can get to it easily, but be careful or you'll cause bleeding, not to mention a lot of discomfort.

Another method is to dab some glue on a cotton swab and touch the glue to the foreign object. If you use this method, be careful not to get the glue on the nasal lining.

Usually the easiest way to get something out of your nose is to hold the unaffected nostril closed and blow. But young children, who are the usual suspects when it comes to foreign bodies in the nose, may not have figured out how to do this effectively. And that's when a "mother's kiss" can come in oh so handy (see below).

Mother's Kiss

The name of this procedure comes from a little trick: to ease the child's anxiety, tell him he's about to get a big kiss.

1. Seal your mouth over the child's open mouth.

2. Press the unaffected nostril shut.

3. Blow until you feel resistance. That's your clue that the glottis is sealing the opening to the lungs, the same way it does when we swallow.

4. When you feel that resistance, blow sharply. One puff, maybe two, should do it.

Studies have found that this works about 60 percent of the time.

7

HEART TO HEART

POP QUIZ

While I was in training at a large urban hospital, a doctor told me about a man who'd come into the emergency room the night before. He was pale, his blood pressure was down, and his heart was racing. The treatment and recovery were uneventful, but the tale he told was unique. He said he was driving down the interstate, passing through to another destination, when he felt his heart rate kick into overdrive.

"Doc, I've got to be the luckiest man around. I've had this heart-racing thing before, and the only thing I've found to cure it is to stand on my head. Well, when it started up tonight, I pulled over and started to do just that. But suddenly, I saw a miracle. Right there, with my head upside down, between my legs, I spotted this hospital. I knew this was the place to come, and here I am."

I'm not making this up. But was he? True or false:

A. This heart problem always has a known trigger—that makes it begin.

B. Before even examining this man, it's possible to guess his problem just by hearing his story.

C. There are other methods that sound about as weird but work as well or better for this type of heart problem.

D. Although the problem seems worrisome, it's not dangerous.

ANSWERS

A. False. Many times the cause is unknown, and it can start for no known reason.

B. True. Supraventricular tachycardia (SVT) is the only heart problem, at least that I know of, that standing on your head can stop. With SVT, electrical signals bypass the area of the heart that normally controls the rate. Another area takes over that likes to keep the rate right around 150 beats per minute. (The normal rate is 60 to 100 beats per minute.)

C. True. There are several other methods, such as gagging yourself or throwing a cold towel on your face, that can stop SVT. Without a way to make a proper diagnosis, and when expert help not an option, you might just have to try it and see if it works.

D. False. Besides the fact that it's overworked, the heart can't pump efficiently at that many beats per minute. If the heart is already weak or there's poor circulation, SVT could make it a lot worse.

CHEST PAIN

When someone has chest pain, the first thought—the biggest worry—is usually a heart attack. Sometimes it can be hard to tell whether that's the problem even in a hospital setting. If you're worried, don't take chances. Call 911 if you can.

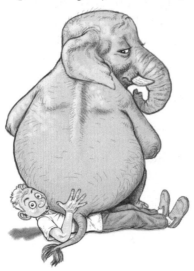

CLASSIC HEART ATTACK SYMPTOMS

Classic heart attack symptoms include a squeezing or crushing type of pain in the middle of the chest that lasts at least several minutes, along with shortness of breath, nausea, and sweating. Pain or a tingling sensation radiates down the left arm, below the elbow, or into the jaw.

But the problem is that many heart attacks aren't classic. Some people have only shortness of breath, nausea, heart palpitations, or just a feeling of fatigue. Yeah, who doesn't have those occasionally, right? So let's look at some other clues to pay attention to.

Risk Factors

Anything that puts you at higher risk of a heart attack than normal should make your worry meter rise when you have suspicious symptoms. Risk factors include known heart problems, family history, high cholesterol, diabetes, and high blood pressure that's not well controlled. Smoking, being overweight, and being inactive also increase your odds. Age is a factor, too: risk increases at age thirty-five and older, and the odds are greatest at sixty-five and older.

However, some people with no known risk factors have heart attacks, so if you have concerns, err on the safe side and get help if you can.

Treatment

First steps:

1. Unless you're absolutely sure the chest pain is not coming from your heart, call 911. Don't hesitate. Seconds may count, and an ambulance will have lifesaving equipment and expert help that's not available in your car. Still, if 911 is not available, being driven to a hospital may be your next best option.

2. Chew up and swallow an aspirin. (Chewing theoretically gets the medicine into your bloodstream quicker, because part of it melts in your mouth and goes through the mucous membranes.) It could help keep the clot in your artery that's causing the heart attack from getting worse. A baby aspirin is enough, but any size works.

3. Lie down, and try your best to relax. I know the relaxing part is asking a lot, but you want to put as little physical and mental stress on your heart as you can.

4. If you're in a public place, have someone locate the nearest automated external defibrillator (AED), just in case your heart goes into a non-life-sustaining rhythm—i.e., you collapse and require CPR.

Then, if you can't get expert help:

- Take in as much oxygen as you can. If you have a canister, use it. If you don't, have someone open a window (unless it's very cold outside; see below). Don't smoke or have smoke in the air you're breathing.

HEART TO HEART

- Try to stay warm. Use a blanket if necessary. If you're cold, the body doesn't function as well as it does when it's warm, and it has to use more energy.

- Use whatever medicine you have available for pain.

- Rest. Bed rest is very important to put less stress on the heart. This should go on for weeks, to give the heart time to heal, but that's obviously pretty impractical, so I'd rest completely for three days if possible or at least for twenty-four hours after the pain goes away. After that, start sitting up for meals and going to the bathroom.

- Don't do strenuous exercise for at least six weeks.

- Continue an aspirin a day indefinitely unless you have a blood disorder or ulcers or are on warfarin (Coumadin).

- See a doctor as soon as you can.

Automated External Defibrillator

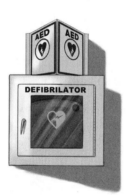

Sometimes when a heart stops beating, rather than becoming completely still, the heart muscle just quivers. The electrical system that makes it beat is still there, it's just not working correctly. This condition is called ventricular fibrillation (V-fib).

The sooner the heart can be shocked with a medical defibrillator, the better the chances of its reverting back into a normal rhythm. One of the main reasons to do chest compressions is to keep the blood flowing to the brain until this shock can be performed.

A defibrillator used to be available only to medical professionals, but now you can often find one on in public places. Look for the letters AED on a box on the wall. All you have to do is open the box and turn on the machine. A computerized voice will walk you through the steps. It will tell you where to place the pads, and the machine will check whether the heart is in V-fib or in another rhythm. If the machine deems that the heart needs a shock, it'll tell you to push a button to charge the device and then to stand back as you push a button to deliver the shock.

OTHER CAUSES OF CHEST PAIN

Chest pain almost always comes from one of four places:

1. The chest wall (ribs, spine, and muscles)—examples include muscle strain and costochondritis (inflammation in some rib joints)

2. The heart or the blood vessels—examples include angina, myocarditis (inflammation of a heart muscle), and a dissecting aneurysm (a tear in the aorta, a major artery)

3. The lungs or the lining of the lungs—examples include pleurisy (inflammation of the lung lining), pneumonia, a pulmonary embolism (blockage of an artery in the lungs), and pneumothorax (a collapsed lung)

4. The esophagus—examples include indigestion (heartburn)

A muscle strain is something you'd treat like any other strain—with heat, rest, and an NSAID (a nonsteroidal anti-inflammatory drug, such as aspirin, Advil, or Aleve). A dissecting aneurysm requires immediate expert care and possible surgery. Minutes can make the difference.

Costochondritis

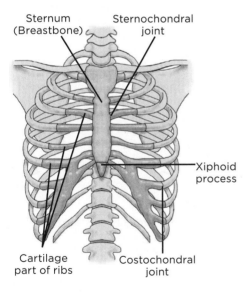

Sternum (Breastbone)

Sternochondral joint

Xiphoid process

Cartilage part of ribs

Costochondral joint

The first few inches of your ribs, starting from where they connect to your breastbone and extending outward to the sides, are made of cartilage. At around the nipple line the cartilage part connects to the bony rib. Both of these connections, or joints, usually only move ever so slightly. But like any joint, they can become inflamed—even sprained—and painful. Possible causes of this inflammation include repetitive pushing and pulling, having a chronic cough, and having large breasts.

One clue that you may have costochondritis is chest pain in those rib-joint areas that worsens with deep breaths or arm movements. Pressing on the joint area also makes the pain worse.

Taking an anti-inflammatory, such as ibuprofen (Advil) or naproxen (Aleve), can help with the pain, as can using a heating pad set to a moderate temperature or applying warm towels to the area for about twenty minutes every two to four hours. Avoid the activity you think caused the pain. If you have large breasts, wear a good full-support bra.

If the pain is severe, a doctor can inject the joint with an anesthetic (a numbing medicine) for temporary relief. Sometimes a steroid injection is added for longer-lasting relief.

Angina

Angina pectoris, or angina for short, could be thought of as a temporary or reversible heart attack. It affects the same heart arteries that, when blocked, cause a heart attack. Angina is dangerous and needs to be recognized as soon as possible and treated by experts once you can get to them.

When you have angina, the arteries are narrowed, usually by fatty plaques (a condition called atherosclerosis), instead of fully blocked. They're narrowed so much that sometimes they can't supply the heart muscle with enough blood.

The anginal pain is the heart's way of saying, "Help! I'm dying here." You might suspect angina if the chest pain is brought on by exercise and goes away in less than five minutes with rest. If it doesn't, you may be having a heart attack.

If you haven't had the symptoms of angina before, treat it like a heart attack. Call 911 if you can.

If you know you have angina and you've been evaluated, follow your doctor's orders, including recommendations for lifestyle changes and symptoms to look for that mean you should get emergency help. If possible, call 911 if the pain is more prolonged than your usual angina episodes.

There are many medicines that can treat angina by helping increase blood flow and decrease the workload on your heart. These include nitroglycerin, aspirin, clot-preventing drugs such as clopidogrel (Plavix), beta-blockers, calcium channel blockers, and other blood-pressure-lowering medicines.

Supplemental oxygen, as needed, can also help. Stay away from smoke.

Angina of the Legs

Intermittent claudication, or angina of the legs, follows the same principle as angina pectoris (pectoris means chest) except that it involves the leg muscles and the arteries nourishing them. If you have this disorder, a certain level of walking brings on leg pain. Stopping relieves it.

There are prescription medicines that help. For various reasons, nitroglycerin and some of the other medicines that treat angina pectoris just don't do as much for the leg arteries. The supplement ginkgo biloba has shown promise in a few studies. Sometimes surgery is the answer, because if the artery clogs completely, you could lose a foot or leg. Smoking is a big risk factor.

BLOOD PRESSURE

First things first. Blood pressure is a good thing. If you don't have any, you're dead. In a survival situation you want to check blood pressure in anyone with dizziness, trauma, fever, a bad headache, a nosebleed, or possible dehydration and almost always as a routine measure if you're checking for any medical problem and a cuff is available.

The general consensus is that 120/80 is a normal blood pressure. Even a little above that increases your long-term risk of heart disease. If the systolic reading (the first number) gets to, say, around 180–200, or the diastolic reading (the second number) gets to 120 or more, it becomes a very real and immediate threat to the heart and brain—possibly leading to a heart attack or stroke.

On the other hand, a reading below 120/80 can be normal and even healthy for some people. As long as it's not out of the ordinary for them; they feel okay; and there's no sign of anemia, dehydration, or a weakened heart, for example, even something like 90/60 can be okay. But sometimes it's not. So how can you tell?

A good rule of thumb is if the blood pressure is low and the person is alert, ask what her usual reading is. Next, check the pulse. If it's over 100, that can be a sign of dehydration or blood loss, perhaps from a wound you haven't found or from internal bleeding. A pulse under 60 could mean that the low blood pressure is from some sort of heart problem or something neurological, such as a stroke. Or the person could be on a beta-blocker heart medication. Also, long-distance runners and cyclists can have normal pulses below 60.

But no matter the pulse, any blood pressure below 90/60 or that has dropped more than thirty points from normal is an indication of serious problems and needs immediate expert attention if possible to find and treat the underlying cause.

In the meantime, lying down can help. IV fluids are a common treatment.

HOW TO CHECK BLOOD PRESSURE

Consider keeping a blood pressure cuff with your first aid supplies. An automatic cuff is easier to use and convenient for routine home checks (which are a good idea if you have high blood pressure). But a manual one works without batteries, is lighter to pack, and can double as a tourniquet.

Here's how to use a manual cuff:

1. Put the cuff around the person's upper arm (or wrist, depending on the type of cuff).

2. Pump air into the cuff using the attached balloon. Watch the needle on the gauge as you pump. If the needle is not going up, you may need to twist the little knob on the tubing next to the balloon to make sure it's in the correct position. It should be turned so that it shuts off any air trying to escape once you've pumped it in.

3. When the needle stops bouncing back and forth, you've cut off blood supply. (The cuff has become a tourniquet.) Stop pumping.

4. If you have a stethoscope, hold it on the person's inner elbow to get ready to listen for the pulse.

5. Twist the silver knob on the balloon a little to slowly let the air out.

6. While watching the gauge, listen with the stethoscope for the first thump of the heart beating. The gauge pressure at that point is the systolic reading—the 120 in 120/80. (That's the pressure at which the blood is first able to squirt through. It's the highest pressure the artery wall gets. It happens when the heart is in a beat.)

7. As more air is let out, the thump will disappear. That's when the cuff's pressure reaches a point where all the blood is going through all the time. That's the diastolic reading—the 80 in 120/80. (It's the lowest pressure the artery wall gets; it happens between heartbeats.)

If you don't have a stethoscope, feel for the radial pulse (in the wrist) as you let the cuff pressure down. When you detect a pulse, that's the systolic reading. You can't check the diastolic pressure this way, but you can get a general idea of whether the systolic is extremely low or high. This method may be your best option when there's a lot of movement and noise, or if the blood pressure is so low that an automatic cuff can't pick it up.

DRUG-FREE TREATMENTS FOR HIGH BLOOD PRESSURE

If you have chronic high blood pressure (hypertension), prescription medication can be a lifesaver. If you can't get to your meds in a survival situation, here are some things may help:

- Cutting back on high-sodium foods and beverages

- Eating potassium-rich foods (if your hypertension hasn't caused kidney damage, which can be detected by routine blood tests)

- Taking magnesium and calcium supplements

Supplements That May Help the Heart

When your heart is weak and prescription medicine is impossible to get, these supplements just might keep you going. But in normal situations, ask your doctor before taking any of them, and read up on dosages, interactions, and side effects, because these supplements are far from perfect. On occasion, they make some people worse or interfere with what they're already taking.

- **L-carnitine** has shown promise in treating angina, intermittent claudication (angina of the legs), and congestive heart failure. The dosage is 1,000 milligrams three times a day. However, some studies have suggested that taking it for more than a year might actually increase your risk of heart disease.

- **Hawthorn extract** can help the heart pump a bit more strongly, widen arteries to increase blood flow, and lower blood pressure. Regarding heart problems, it's been shown to be most effective in treating mild congestive heart failure. But sometimes it can make symptoms worse. And it can have bad interactions with other heart medicines. You should take it only under a physician's supervision. The dosage ranges from 250 milligrams to 100 milligrams twice a day.

- **Coenzyme Q10** can lower blood pressure and help treat congestive heart failure. Don't take it if you're pregnant or taking a prescription blood thinner such as warfarin (Coumadin). The dosage is 50 to 100 milligrams twice a day.

- **Fish oil** has omega-3 fatty acids that can lower your level of triglycerides (a type of bad cholesterol), increase levels of HDL cholesterol (the good type), help minimize inflammation and blood clotting, and keep blood vessels healthy.

- Eating a clove (segment) or two of raw garlic daily, which may lower blood pressure 7–8 percent or so

- Getting enough vitamins D and C (deficiencies can raise blood pressure)

- Avoiding over-the-counter medicines and nasal sprays unless the labeled precautions don't list a possible effect on blood pressure

- Losing weight if you're overweight

- Getting regular, moderate exercise (check with your doctor before starting a vigorous program)

Before you get into a survival situation, ask your doctor about incorporating some of these things now to try to reduce your need for medication.

If you don't think you have high blood pressure but haven't been checked within the last year, get to a clinic to make sure. Hypertension usually has no symptoms; it just does its damage to your heart and blood vessels silently.

FAST HEART RATE

A normal heart rate is 60 to 100 (a bit lower for some athletes). If it's going at a speed of 100–110 and it's at a regular rhythm (maybe a few skips), you could be just overtired or nervous. Sit or lie down for a few minutes and try to relax. Dehydration, fever, and anemia can cause the heart to beat fast like this also. The rate should lower when you treat the underlying cause. Of course, exercise can cause the rate to temporarily be much higher.

If a fast heart rate is caused directly by heart problems, many times there's not much to do in the field except have the person rest. Paroxysmal supraventricular tachycardia is an exception.

PAROXYSMAL SUPRAVENTRICULAR TACHYCARDIA (PSVT)

The heart sends and receives electrical signals that are all synchronized to ensure that blood is pumped to the body effectively. When those signals get messed up, the heart beats abnormally and isn't able to do its job as well.

There are various types of abnormal heart rates that are caused by such signal malfunctions. But for one in particular—paroxysmal supraventricular tachycardia, or PSVT—there are some tricks you can try to fix it even if expert care is impossible. ("Paroxysmal" means it comes and goes. "Tachycardia" means "fast heartbeat." "Supraventricular" indicates where the problem starts—above the ventricles.)

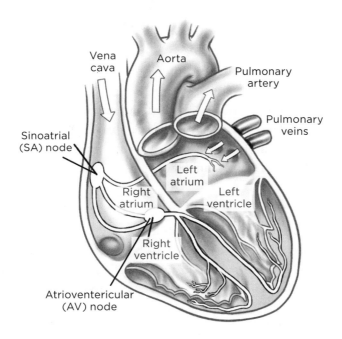

Fast Check for a Fast Heart Rate

Heart rate is measured in beats per minute. If you have a watch with a second hand, count the heartbeats for ten seconds and then multiply by six. Or count the beats for fifteen seconds and multiply by four.

If you don't have a watch, hum the song "Stayin' Alive" or "Another One Bites the Dust" while taking the pulse. The tempo of both tunes is about 100 beats per minute, so if the heart beats a lot faster than the songs, you know you're dealing with a fast heart rate.

You can also practice in advance to get a feel for a normal rate. Check your pulse both with and without counting, so if you don't have a watch when you need it, you can discern when the rate is way too fast. For a recap on how to check a pulse, see page 39.

Clues

PSVT usually causes a heartbeat of around 150–180, sometimes higher. Symptoms can range from a feeling of the heart racing or a chest tightness to no symptoms at all. Dizziness is common. There are other types of SVTs with similar symptoms and rates, all treated with medicines or medical procedures, but unlike them, PSVT is more likely to just start out of the blue and stop the same way (hence its designation as "paroxysmal"). And it's the only SVT that the vagal maneuvers described below will sometimes stop.

Causes

Thyroid disease can cause PSVT, as can certain prescription medications, smoking, anxiety, recreational drugs, and a condition called Wolff-Parkinson-White syndrome (a slight electrical-system abnormality that some people are born with). Often, though, the cause remains unknown.

Dangers

Because the heart can't pump blood efficiently during an episode of PSVT, it can become overworked if the problem goes untreated. A healthy heart can withstand this for a while without permanent injury, but PSVT can be especially dangerous if the heart is already burdened by narrow arteries (atherosclerosis), congestive heart failure, or lung problems that keep the blood from getting enough oxygen.

Treatment

There are prescription medicines that treat PSVT and some that can help prevent it. But until you can get medical help, there are a few things you can do to try to kick your heart rate back to normal. All these are called vagal maneuvers. The vagus nerve, which runs from the brainstem to the abdomen, is a major nerve that, among many other functions, helps control heart rate.

Valsalva maneuver: Hold your breath and bear down in a strain, as if you're constipated and straining to have a bowel movement. Do this for five seconds, then breathe. This changes the pressure in your chest and therefore in the big blood vessels in it. Your body gets fooled into thinking your heart should slow down. If the pulse doesn't slow, try again.

Another way to do the Valsalva maneuver is to stick a finger in your throat and gag yourself. Or pinch your nostrils, close your mouth, and exhale, as if you were trying to equalize the pressure in your ears. A few coughs can also be worth a try.

Ice-water facial: If you have access to ice water or even cold water, dip your face in it for a few seconds. Or just slap on an ice bag or cold cloth. This stimulates your vagus nerve to slow your heart by causing what's known as the dive reflex. It's the same reflex that allows some children to survive for many minutes under cold water without brain damage.

Carotid maneuver: This should actually be done at the doctor's office because of the possible side effects, such as a temporary but really fast lowering of blood pressure.

Lie down and find your carotid pulse just below your jaw. There are some very sensitive nerve fibers there. Massage firmly for five seconds. This can reset a fast heart rate into a normal one, even if the tachycardia is caused by something other than PSVT. If you have one of those other conditions, though, the heart rate goes back up as soon as you stop the massage.

Warning: In rare cases the carotid maneuver could knock off a piece of a blood clot lodged in the neck and cause a stroke. Don't perform it on older people—around sixty-five and up—or anyone with a history of stroke. It can also cause fainting if it causes the heart to skip a few beats or if the blood pressure goes down quickly.

Headstand: And then, as in the story at the beginning of this chapter (page 125), there the few people who swear that standing on your head for thirty seconds is the only way to go.

Prevention

To try to prevent PSVT from coming back, don't use tobacco, caffeine, or alcohol. Get regular exercise. And limit stress or try meditation, biofeedback, or other calming alternatives.

PANIC ATTACK

A panic attack can feel just like a heart attack and just as frightening. In fact, it's hard to convince some people who are having a panic attack that it's not their heart, because the symptoms are so scary.

We're not sure what causes panic attacks, but we think it has to do with your body going into fight-or-flight mode, sometimes for no specific reason. And it seems that some people's bodies have a lower trigger point for this than others.

We do know that even if you're getting plenty of oxygen, if the level of carbon dioxide in your blood lowers past a certain threshold, you get short of breath. Some studies have found that people prone to panic attacks breathe a little differently, which keeps their carbon dioxide at a constant low level, close to that threshold.

CLUES

A panic attack may cause:

- Tingling of the fingers, toes, or face
- Muscle cramping in the hands or feet
- Chest tightness
- A feeling of impending doom

The pulse rate may be high, but probably not over 120. The blood oxygen level is normal. A pulse oximeter (see page 152) is a little device sold over the counter that slips onto your fingertip and measures the oxygen in your blood. When you're having a panic attack, even though you feel like you're starving for air, a pulse oximeter will show that your blood oxygen level is at or close to 100 percent.

The only way to truly rule out heart and lung problems if you're having symptoms of a heart attack is to undergo a series of tests in a medical facility.

TREATMENT

Concentrate on taking in slow breaths, preferably through your nose. Take about six to eight seconds to blow out through your pursed lips (puckered as if you're going to whistle). Try to use your abdomen by expanding it as you breathe in. Putting a hand on your belly can help you focus on doing this. In a panic attack, once you start breathing fast, you lose more carbon dioxide than normal. That creates a lot of your symptoms, including the intense feeling that you need more air. Gulping for the air makes you lose more carbon dioxide, which makes you more short of breath, perpetuating the cycle..

If the slow abdominal breathing isn't working, consider doing it while breathing into a paper bag. Of course, if you have lung disease, this may not be such a great idea, because you'd be getting less oxygen than you would otherwise. (Exhaled air contains an average of 17 percent oxygen, as opposed to the 21 percent you get when you inhale.) But for those of us without lung disease, exhaled air provides plenty of oxygen. If the bag hasn't helped in a minute or two, you should start thinking of heart and lung problems that may be causing your symptoms.

Medications for anxiety can also help.

PREVENTION

Different prevention methods work for different people. These are some with a good track record:

- Antidepressants in the SSRI family (selective serotonin reuptake inhibitors), such as Celexa, Paxil, Prozac, and Zoloft

- Treatment for any underlying anxiety

- A relaxation technique, such as proper breathing or meditation

- Quitting tobacco use

- Limiting caffeine intake

- Taking zinc and magnesium supplements

BLOOD CLOTS IN THE LEGS

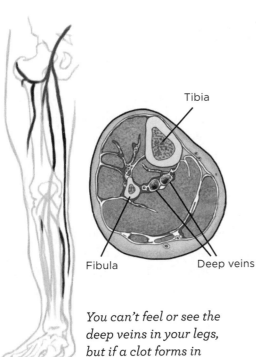

Tibia

Fibula   Deep veins

You can't feel or see the deep veins in your legs, but if a clot forms in one, it can sometimes be painful and is always potentially dangerous.

Most people I see with blood clots in their legs have the relatively harmless kind that lodges in the soft tissue or muscle. They've bumped a leg and feel a knot. This isn't dangerous.

If a clot has formed in a deep vein, though, it is dangerous. It's called deep vein thrombosis. Most of the time these clots are too deep to feel, but sometimes the calf is swollen and tender all over, and it hurts to flex the ankle, bringing the toes upward.

Some of the many causes of deep vein thrombosis are trauma, certain medications, and being sedentary. The danger is that a tiny piece of that clot might break off and head for your lungs. This can be deadly, and it's why anyone with signs of this clot needs medical attention ASAP.

If you suspect deep vein thrombosis and proper medical care is impossible, get off your feet. Keep the leg elevated at heart level or above. Apply heat, if available, for twenty minutes every two hours or so. The heat can come in the form of hot water bottles or warm, moist towels. Do this until emergency personnel can get to you.

Nothing can take the place of prescription blood thinners to keep these clots from expanding, but if it's going to be weeks before you can get proper medical help, it's worth a try to take a baby aspirin or half of an adult aspirin daily if you're not allergic and have no history of bleeding problems or stomach ulcers.

A blood clot can also form in a superficial vessel, often a varicose vein (a vein that usually pokes out because its valves don't work well, allowing blood to pool inside it). The area around the clot can get inflamed (red, painful, and swollen). People usually feel a localized area of tenderness rather than a sore calf. Treatment is the same as above, but there's no urgent threat to your life. Still, see a doctor as soon as possible. What you think is a superficial clot may be deep vein thrombosis: even the experts can be fooled without special testing.

BLOOD CLOTS IN THE LUNGS

Sometimes a blood clot in a deep leg vein can flick off a small piece of clotted material that travels to the heart. The heart then pumps this small clot (called an embolus) into a blood vessel in one of the lungs, cutting off the blood supply to this area of the lung. This condition, called a pulmonary embolism, can cause a chain reaction of dead lung tissue and swelling and is very dangerous.

CLUES

If you have a pulmonary embolism, breathing will be painful, and you may become very short of breath. One of your calves may be sore and swollen—it may have been beforehand, too—and this could be where the clot came from. But often, there is no warning. Blood clots can be very hard to diagnose without specialized testing.

TREATMENT

You need transfer to a medical facility if at all possible if you have any suspicion that there may be an embolus or if there's no other explanation for your shortness of breath that can be resolved with treatment in the field. Many people with a pulmonary embolism die within the first few hours after the clot breaks off. Early treatment is essential.

You may be prescribed bed rest and blood thinners to prevent additional clots. Some people will be given medicines called clot busters to dissolve the clot quickly. Oxygen and close observation in intensive care are usually needed.

CARDIOPULMONARY RESUSCITATION (CPR)

On TV—the only place many people have seen CPR performed—the actors still do chest compressions plus artificial respiration. Hollywood hasn't caught up to the latest guidelines.

Since 2008, unless you're an expert at doing artificial respiration, the recommendation has been to concentrate on doing really good chest compressions in most situations (for exceptions to this rule, see page 164).

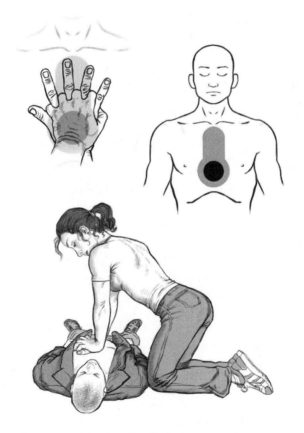

Proper positioning for chest compressions

Before you start CPR, make sure the victim needs it—that she has no signs of life. Yell; pinch the shoulder or face to try to get a response; watch the chest for breathing. Your first thought may be to check for a pulse. The risk is that you could waste a lot of time trying to find it—or you could mistake your own pulse, which is probably strong from the excitement, for the victim's. (If there are signs of life, she does not need CPR, but she may need treatment. Consider going through your AEIOU TIPS, page 73.)

If you're in a public building or anywhere else where you think there might be an automatic external defibrillator, have someone try to find it immediately. It might be labeled AED (see page 128). If you're the only person around, don't take more than about thirty seconds to look for one.

Do all this quickly, because the sooner you start chest compressions on someone whose heart has stopped the better. Of course, all the while, yell for help, and, if you're able to, call 911.

Then, ensure that the person is on her back lying on a firm surface. The following instructions are applicable if the victim is an adult or an older child. For small children and babies, see page 143.

1. Kneel next to the chest (assuming the victim is on the floor).

2. Locate the center of the breastbone at a level that's between the nipples.

3. Lean over the victim, with your shoulders directly over that centered point, and place the heel of one of your hands at that point.

4. Place the heel of your other hand on top of the first, and intertwine the fingers of your two hands.

5. With your arms outstretched and elbows locked, use your body weight to push down deep and fast. The chest should compress about two inches (about one-third the depth of the chest). Then let off the pressure to allow it to rise back fully. Keep your elbows locked even when you're not pushing down.

6. Repeat step five at the rate of one hundred compressions per minute. As when you're taking a pulse (see page 39), one trick for estimating the right speed is to sing the Bee Gees song "Stayin' Alive" or the Queen song "Another One Bites the Dust" in your head as you do the compressions.

If at some point an AED machine arrives, have someone immediately open it and turn it on. Follow the verbal directions.

Until expert help arrives or you're exhausted, never stop compressions except for the few seconds when the AED says "Clear" or "Stand back." Since it's virtually impossible for one person to continue adequate chest compressions for more than a couple of minutes at a time, try to recruit help.

It's rare for CPR alone to revive a victim. Its main purpose is to keep oxygen-giving blood circulating to the brain until experts, with all their specialized machines and medicines, can take over.

CPR FOR BABIES AND SMALL CHILDREN

When the victim is a small child, pushing on the midchest with one hand rather than two will probably effectively compress the chest. For a baby, use two fingers instead of a hand. And rather than place the baby on the floor, you could hold him in the position shown for compressions on page 163.

For small children and babies, the compression rate is the same as for adults. A big difference, however, is that artificial respirations (see page 164) are as important for these youngsters as compressions. That's because choking or a lung problem is much more likely the reason for collapse than a heart problem. For adults it's just the opposite.

So compress the chest about one-third of its depth 30 times. Give two breaths, and repeat.

Precordial Thump

Experts used to recommend trying a precordial thump before starting chest compressions. That's one sharp hit on the middle of the chest to try to shock the heart into returning to a normal beat—similar to what the manual defibrillator does, though it uses electricity instead of force. Since the precordial thump is rarely if ever effective, it's now thought to be a waste of time. But in a situation where there's no AED and help is not coming, one thump might be worth a try.

8

JUST BREATHE

POP QUIZ

Years ago, I was talking to a patient in the emergency room when one of the nurses tapped me on the shoulder. She was grimacing and holding the side of her chest.

"I think I have a collapsed lung."

She was breathing a tad heavily, but nothing like the people I'd seen with a collapsed lung in the past. I was a little dubious. "Why do you think that?" I asked.

"I've had one—actually two—before."

"Oh?" I turned around. "What are your symptoms?"

"I was feeling fine, and out of the blue, I began having this really bad pain in my chest, worse when I take a deep breath?"

Sure enough, when I listened to her chest, the breath sounds on one side were weaker than on the other. What do you think I did after that?

A. Had her lie back, numbed up a spot, and stuck a needle in her chest to suck out the air that had been released from her lung, thus relieving the pressure.

B. Checked her blood oxygen level and ordered a chest X-ray, then stuck the needle in.

C. Inserted a chest tube, attached it to a suction machine, and admitted her to the hospital for monitoring.

D. Admitted her to the hospital to monitor, gave her some anti-inflammatories for pain, and that's about it.

ANSWERS

A. Incorrect. A needle can have serious side effects. It's rare, but it could have punctured a blood vessel or the lung lining or created a wound where an infection could develop.

B. Incorrect. I did check her blood oxygen level right away, which was normal, and a subsequent chest X-ray showed that the collapse was only partial, but even if those tests hadn't been available to support my plan, I would have opted for a conservative treatment. Why? Because I was not only treating a diagnosis, I was also treating a specific person. She was mildly short of breath at worst. So first do not harm, right? Of course, I had the oxygen level to back me up and the knowledge that a spontaneous pneumothorax like this one typically heals on its own.

C. Incorrect. Like a needle, a chest tube can have serious side effects, so it's best to avoid it if possible.

D. Correct. Believe or not, I chose D. First, since there had been no trauma and there were no chest wounds, I surmised that her lung had sprung a leak from the inside, possibly from the place it had in the past (once you have one spontaneous leak, you're at risk for another), or she might have a bleb, a.k.a. a lung blister. That's a little bubbled-up weak spot that leaks easily. Some people are born with a few of them. When one bursts, the air seeps out between the lung and the chest wall, and the lung starts collapsing because that air, now trapped inside the chest wall, is taking up part of the space that the lung usually occupies. The more air, the more the collapse. Sometimes the lung fully collapses; sometimes the air pressure on both sides equalizes and it collapses partially. In that case the lung is still functioning, just not as well as it does normally.

It would have been a whole different matter if she'd been extremely short of breath. Then I might have tried to suck the air out to see if that helped. Usually, though, the area will fill right back up after that, so I would have then inserted a chest tube connected to constant suction. Over a few days, the lung lining would heal and seal over and I could take the tube out.

Lot of ifs, huh? Many times we have to make judgment calls depending on whatever knowledge we can glean about a situation, what's available to work with, and our assessment of what has to be done to save a life. Then we weigh the potential complications versus benefits of a given treatment.

So in the nurse's case we waited and watched to make sure her symptoms didn't get worse. She had periodic X-rays to make sure the pneumothorax wasn't expanding. After a day, she went home to rest. In a few weeks the leak healed, the air absorbed into her body tissues, her lung expanded back to its normal size, and she got back to work.

Lungs

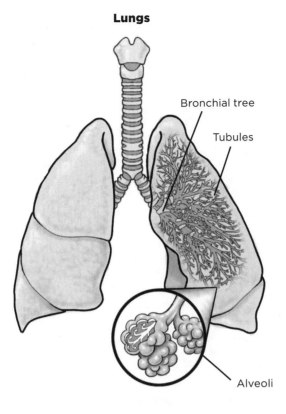

Bronchial tree

Tubules

Alveoli

WHY WE LOVE OUR LUNGS

Don't you just love breathing in fresh air—taking time to savor it? It brings an almost automatic smile. There's a biological reason for that, of course. Fresh air is your best natural source of life-giving oxygen.

Your lungs have two main functions:

1. They transport oxygen to your arteries. The arteries then transport it to every cell in your body.

2. They remove carbon dioxide from your blood and get rid of it when you exhale.

You could think of the lungs as two sophisticated bags, airtight except for a single opening that starts at the nose and mouth, becomes the trachea, and branches into two bronchial tubes, one entering each lung. These tubes then branch into smaller and smaller bronchial tubes. The smallest branches are called bronchioles. Every lung has thousands of them. Finally, each bronchiole ends in several tiny, saclike alveoli. The walls of an alveolus are where the oxygen-and-carbon-dioxide exchange takes place.

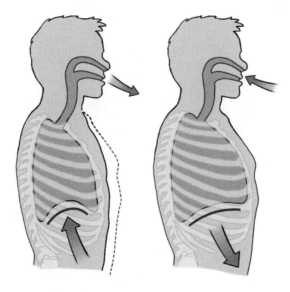

The chest cavity contracts to push air out and expands to pull air in.

NATURE ABHORS A VACUUM

If you remember science class, you know that when I say "vacuum," I'm not talking about a rug cleaner. In science lingo, a vacuum is a space with nothing in it. No air, water—nada. And on Earth, that's just not normal, at least for long. If there's any opening at all to that vacuum, something is going to find its way in. A fireplace bellows is a simple example. Expand it, and air rushes in to fill the new space.

Your lungs work in a similar way. When you inhale, your diaphragm—the muscle that separates your chest cavity from your abdomen—contracts and flattens. At the same time, other muscles expand the chest wall. All this makes the cavity expand, like the bellows. This creates a new space (vacuum), and air rushes in through your mouth and nose. When you exhale, the opposite happens: the chest space is made smaller, and air is pushed out. A puncture in the chest wall can break the vacuum seal and stop this smooth cycle (see page 151).

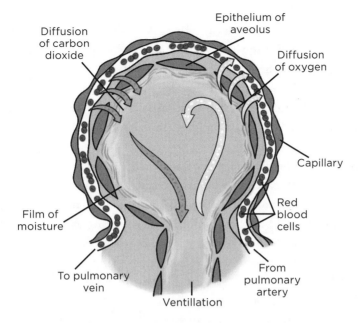

The alveolus is where oxygen diffuses from the lung into the blood and carbon dioxide comes out from the blood into the lung.

WHAT EXTREME BREATH RATES TELL YOU

When you're at rest, twelve to sixteen breaths per minute gives you enough oxygen while keeping the carbon dioxide in your blood in a normal range. You breathe a little faster if you're doing manual labor or running a fever or if anything else is increasing your metabolism. But if your breath rate gets too much higher or lower, you need to start looking for a reason.

An extremely high or low breath rate tells you there's an underlying problem that needs to be addressed—soon. Otherwise, your body may give out, either from exhaustion (with a high rate) or lack of oxygen (with a low rate).

If your respiration rate at rest gets above twenty to twenty-four breaths per minute, your body may be trying to compensate for a reduced ability to pull in oxygen. Potential causes include a collapsed lung, pneumonia, and fluid in or around the lung.

Hyperventilation from a panic attack causes you to breathe fast for a different reason. Your body has been tricked into thinking you need that rate of respiration even though you're getting plenty of oxygen (see page 137).

Whatever the reason, if the breath rate stays around twenty-four or above, your muscles will soon fatigue and your breathing will slow to a dangerous level. And if the high breath rate is the only thing keeping your blood oxygen level high enough for you to survive, like when you have a collapsed lung . . . well, it'd be great to find and treat the cause before your muscles give out. Meanwhile, some supplemental oxygen could sure come in handy. If that's still not enough, you may end up needing to get mechanical ventilation in an intensive care unit, if you can, before your muscles give out completely.

Unless it's from pure fatigue, a respiratory rate below eight breaths per minute usually means that the part of the brain that signals you to breathe is malfunctioning. This is sometimes caused by a stroke, head trauma, drugs, or alcohol. At six breaths per minute and below, it's unlikely you're getting enough oxygen to your cells to sustain life, and you're going to need help either from a ventilator or from someone breathing or pumping air into your lungs manually.

In the end, the reason for an abnormally slow or fast rate must be corrected for the breathing to get back on track. And in general, the slower or faster the rate of breathing, the more urgent the need for correction.

COLLAPSED LUNG

When you get air in between the chest wall and the lung, you have a pneumothorax. The air pushes on the lung, and the lung is left with less or no room to expand. The lung has no option but to partially or fully collapse. A pneumothorax can be caused by an internal injury, such as a broken rib that pokes a hole in the lung; a weak spot in the lung that starts leaking; or an external injury, such as a gunshot or stab wound that perforates the chest cavity.

CLUES

Though a pneumothorax can occur without any apparent trauma, you should especially suspect one in anyone with a bad chest injury. People with a pneumothorax will usually show all these signs:

- Shortness of breath
- Chest pain on the affected side
- A hissing sound from a chest wound or bubbles coming from the fluids around one
- Decreased breath sounds on the affected side

SMALL PNEUMOTHORAX

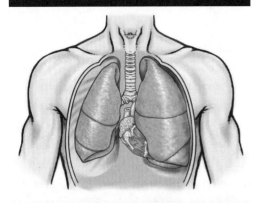

LARGE PNEUMOTHORAX

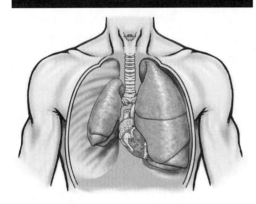

To check for breath sounds, use a stethoscope or put your ear to the back of the victim's chest. Start where the bottom of one lung begins, then compare by listening to the same area of the other lung. Have the victim take deep breaths, and listen throughout. Move up a little and listen to both sides again. Repeat this three or four times until you've listened to both lungs in their entirety. If there is a pneumothorax, the breath sounds will be softer or absent on that side.

A Pneumo with No Wound

It is possible to have a pneumothorax without an external wound. That's called a closed pneumothorax. An injury, such as a broken rib, could cause this, or it can happen spontaneously, as it did to the nurse in the pop quiz on page 145. Usually a person can live with a closed pneumothorax until it heals—unless it develops into a tension pneumo (see page 152).

TREATMENT FOR A SUCKING CHEST WOUND

The lungs adhere to the chest wall with the help of a thin lubricant called surfactant. But let's say you get shot or stabbed in the chest and the wound goes through to the chest cavity. Now, when your chest expands to breathe in, air rushes in not only through your trachea but also through that hole between the chest cavity and the lung, crowding and pressing on the lung. This injury is called a sucking chest wound. To treat it, you'll need to seal the wound so air doesn't keep getting in. Simple. But there's a catch: air that's already built up inside the chest also needs to be able to escape. So how do you make a seal that doesn't let air in but does allow it out?

You use petroleum jelly and gauze.

Coat the gauze with the jelly, and lay your high-tech creation onto the wound.

The jelly will help the gauze stick, but when the person breathes out, the air can push the gauze up a little and escape. Sticking three sides down with tape could help keep it in place.

Or you could take a plain old plastic card from your wallet (such as a credit or ID card) and plop it on the wound. That's all. The blood from the wound should cause the card to stick to the skin. When the victim breathes in, the card will form a tight seal. When the victim breathes out, the card will be loose enough to allow air that's already in the chest cavity to come out. It's better not to use tape on the card, since it might seal too tightly, but check it frequently to make sure it hasn't moved out of position. (This only works if the wound is smaller than the card. If the hole is too big to be sealed by a card, which would be very unusual, expert help is the victim's only hope.) If you don't have a card, you can use a piece of duct tape, folded with the sticky side in.

People can often live with a pneumothorax for minutes to days, depending on the severity of the collapse and the health of the lungs. However, if the condition develops into a tension pneumothorax, the situation becomes more dire.

✚ HOW TO MEASURE BLOOD OXYGEN LEVEL

A little device called a pulse oximeter, sold over the counter, can tell you how well oxygen is getting to your tissues when you have shortness of breath. In general, the lower the oxygen saturation, the more serious your problem is. If it gets down into the low eighties or below, immediate expert help is essential.

On the other hand, someone who's extremely short of breath but has an oxygen saturation level of around 98 to 100 percent is getting plenty of oxygen, so that tells you he's probably hyperventilating from a panic attack.

TENSION PNEUMOTHORAX

If you suspect someone has a pneumothorax, and she's getting worse quickly or losing consciousness, she could have a tension pneumothorax. This is an immediately life-threatening emergency. The leak has become a one-way valve going the wrong way. It pushes air into the area between the chest wall and the lung but won't let it escape, kind of like when you blow up a balloon and hold the opening between puffs. This puts extreme pressure on the heart and both lungs. The blood pressure drops and the pulse increases. The heart may even stop.

Just as you would for any pneumothorax, seal any chest wounds immediately with the one-way-valve method (see page 151) so at least more air won't be coming in.

Then, if the victim seems like she's going to collapse and help is not coming, take a 14-to-16-gauge needle if you have one—at least 1.5 inches long. If the victim isn't already lying down, do your best to get her into that position. Feel for the rib right below the collarbone, then the next one down. Go out a good two inches from the edge of the breastbone and slowly stick the needle just above that rib. (There are blood vessels and nerves under ribs.) If you have an attached syringe, you'll know you've gone far enough if the syringe starts filling with air on its own. At that point you could disconnect the syringe or take out the plunger so more air can escape. If you don't have a syringe you'll hear a hissing.

A medical needle will have a lip around the base, so it shouldn't slip all the way into the chest. If you're using a tattoo needle, it won't have that lip, so be extremely careful.

ASTHMA

I've heard that an asthma attack feels like you're breathing through a drinking straw. I hope I never know firsthand, because that sounds pretty frightening—and serious. And, of course, it is.

Asthma is a chronic disease in which the lining of the bronchial airways inside the lungs is constantly inflamed. In an asthma attack, the airways quickly become more inflamed and swollen, and the muscles around the bronchial tubes go into a spasm. Hence there's less space for air to get through, and you get that feeling of breathing through a straw.

An asthma attack is caused by some sort of trigger—something that sets it off. It reminds me of the way the leaves of some plants automatically curl up when you touch them. And different people have different triggers—exercise, allergens, anxiety, or a number of other things.

CLUES

An asthma attack causes:

- **Shortness of breath:** unless the victim is having her first attack, she'll recognize the feeling

- **Chest tightness**

- **Coughing**

- **Wheezing:** when air moves back and forth through those too-narrow airways it makes a whistling sound. Since it's going through many different sizes of airway at the same time, the various frequencies all simultaneously sound a bit musical—like someone playing the bagpipes very badly. Sometimes the wheezing can be heard by everyone around, but often a stethoscope or putting an ear to the chest is needed.

A pulse oximeter—that little device you clip onto the finger that indicates oxygen level and pulse rate; see page 152—can measure the oxygen in the blood and give you an idea of how bad an asthma attack is. For instance, if the blood oxygen level is below ninety and falling despite what you're doing, you need to get expert help fast.

PREVENTION

Treatment for an asthma attack may be especially hard to come by in a survival situation. Here are some suggestions to get asthma under control now and keep the attacks to a minimum:

1. **Take prescription medicines:** See a doctor and get on a customized treatment regimen. Not doing so means risking preventable permanent lung damage and possibly your life—even outside of a survival situation.

2. **Maintain a healthful weight, and exercise regularly:** Both diet and exercise have been shown to help prevent attacks. Even if exercise is one of your triggers, being in shape will allow you to exert yourself more before you're breathing fast enough to trigger an attack. One way to stay in shape is to find the types of exercises or sports that don't trigger your attacks. Or try exercising just to the point before early symptoms come on, then gradually do more. Always do this under a doctor's supervision and with your albuterol inhaler at hand.

3. **Eat fruits and vegetables:** Antioxidants in fruits and vegetables can strengthen your immunity, helping you avoid respiratory infections, which can be triggers in some people.

4. **Keep current with flu and pneumonia vaccines.**

5. **Practice breathing techniques:** Learn to breathe in through your nose and out slowly through pursed lips. Focus on using your diaphragm by relax-

ing and expanding your abdominal muscles as you breathe in. (It's the same technique used for treating panic attacks.) Specific techniques sometimes take weeks to learn properly. Check with your health care providers for guidance.

6. **Consider taking dietary supplements:** Some supplements may help prevent flare-ups. Talk to your health care provider if you want to work them into your regimen. Here are some of the more popular ones:

   • Supplements that may decrease asthma-related inflammation: These include fish oil, ginger, turmeric, magnesium, and vitamins D and C

   • Pycnogenol: This may allow some people to decrease the dosages of their asthma medicines (the recommended pycnogenol dosage for children is 0.5 mg per pound of body weight given twice a day)

   • Eucalyptus oil: This can help clear mucus, especially when you're sick. You can put it in a vaporizer. Alternatively, several over-the-counter products that you rub on your skin or inhale are available. A very diluted amount is found in some lozenges. But beware of taking it by mouth except under a doctor's supervision; even a tiny amount can cause dangerous reactions.

There are also shorter-term steps that can help with prevention right away. You can use these during a survival situation or in your everyday life:

1. **Drink plenty of water:** Water keeps the lining of your lungs hydrated.

2. **Use a vaporizer:** Steam can also keep the lining of your lungs hydrated.

3. **Cover your nose and mouth with a scarf or mask when you're in cold weather:** Also cover up when you're around smoke and other air irritants.

4. **Avoid the triggers:** Whatever causes problems for you, try to steer clear of it. If you can't, treat the issue before it causes asthma symptoms.

TRIGGERS

Whatever acts as an asthma trigger for you, try to steer clear of it. Some people have multiple triggers, and others have just one. The list of possible triggers includes:

• Respiratory infections

• Smoke of any type

• Air pollution

- Allergens, such as pollens, pet dander, dust mites, or cockroach droppings

- Certain medications, such as aspirin, beta blockers, ACE (angiotensin-converting enzyme) inhibitors, and antihistamines

- Exercise

- Anxiety

- Acid reflux (heartburn; the chronic type is called gastroesophageal reflux disease, or GERD)

- Mold

TREATMENT

Anyone who has asthma should always have an albuterol inhaler on hand. It's a prescription medicine that opens the airways quickly when you're having an attack. Also get oxygen or fresh air, unless that's where the trigger is. And get to a doctor or call 911 if possible. If the asthma attack is out of the ordinary for you, getting expert medical help, and quickly, could save your life.

If expert help is unavailable or delayed, you could try:

1. **Drinking caffeine:** Coffee and tea both contain a chemical similar to the old asthma medicine theophylline. (These days, better medicine with fewer side effects is available, but theophylline was effective.) Many experts think the amount of caffeine in drinks is too small to do much good, but unless you're particularly sensitive to caffeine, a couple of hot cups of coffee or tea could be worth a try if for nothing else than the soothing steam.

2. **Inhaling steam:** To make a steam tent, fill a bowl with hot water and lean over it (after making sure the steam isn't hot enough to scald). Cover your head and the bowl with a blanket or towel to trap the steam. Or sit in a closed bathroom with the hot water on. Just be sure not to burn yourself.

3. **Taking Sudafed (pseudoephedrine):** If you have no inhaler, this decongestant might help during an attack. Know its potential side effects, such as increasing heart rate and blood pressure and causing urinary problems in anyone with an enlarged prostate.

4. **Using an EpiPen:** Everyone should have this prescription device on hand in case of a life-threatening allergic (anaphylactic) reaction. It works on severe asthma attacks as well.

WHEN THE AIRWAY IS BLOCKED BY THE TONGUE

People don't actually ever swallow their tongues, even during a seizure. But the back of the tongue can block the airway under certain circumstances.

Sometimes the tongue swells due to trauma, infection, or an allergic reaction. More often, when a person is unconscious or close to it (as he would be during or right after a seizure), the tongue relaxes, and gravity causes the back of it to block the airway.

TREATMENT

If you're sure there hasn't been a spine injury, simply turning someone who's lying on his back over on his side can cause the tongue to move out of the way. But if a spine injury can't be ruled out (see page 61), or if the victim needs certain procedures, such as chest compressions, you may not be able to turn him over immediately. In that case, you can use an alternative method to clear the airway.

- **Head tilt:** Tilting the head backward and the chin up can open the airway, but that procedure should never be done if there's any chance of a spine injury.

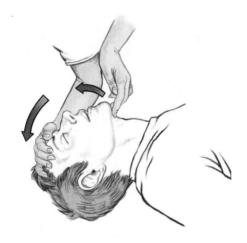

Head tilt

• **Jaw thrust:** This method takes a little practice but shouldn't affect the neck if done properly. Use your index and middle fingers to push the jaw up while your thumbs push down on the chin. It only works well in someone who's unconscious, because then the jaw will be completely relaxed.

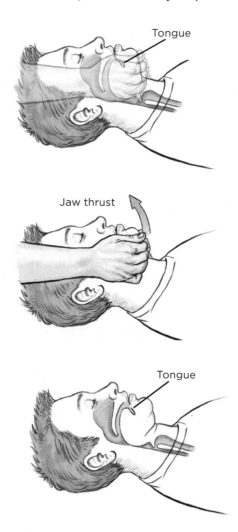

• **Tongue pull:** Find a piece of cloth, grab the tip of the tongue, and pull it forward.

• **Oropharyngeal airway (OPA):** You can buy a package of various sizes of this device and keep it in your first aid kit. Insert the correct size into the airway, and you'll have free hands to continue other procedures. Don't use this in someone who's conscious enough to have a gag reflex. You'll need to know how to properly insert it (see page 159). Never force it, since you could cause injury.

- **Nasopharyngeal airway (NPA):** This device also comes in various sizes. It's inserted through the nose instead of the mouth. It works even if the victim could have a gag reflex. Never force one in. Using a lubricant—preferably water soluble—helps you slide the device in more easily and results in less trauma to the nasal lining. Don't use an NPA if there's been a facial injury around the nose.

✚ HOW TO INSERT AN AIRWAY ADJUNCT

The OPA and NPA are both devices designed to keep the airway opened.

HOW TO INSERT AN OPA

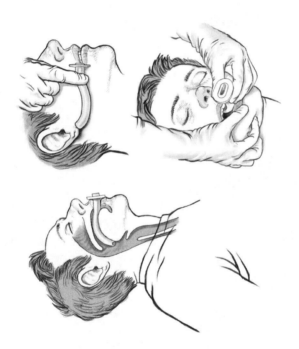

The OPA must be long enough to prevent the base of the tongue from blocking the airway but short enough to not damage things such as the vocal cords. To choose the correct size, place different sizes of OPAs along the side of the face. Choose the one that goes exactly from the corner of the victim's mouth to his earlobe.

The OPA is curved. When first inserting it, the tip should be pointed upward toward the victim's nose so the OPA doesn't push the tongue backward. About halfway in—when you think the tip is close to the back of the mouth—continue inserting the device, but rotate the tube 180 degrees so the tip is pointed toward the lungs. Continue inserting until the flange is at the lips.

Any time you feel resistance—or if for any reason you think you're pushing the tongue backward—pull the OPA completely out and reinsert (tip up, then rotate, as before). If the OPA is in position, air should be passing from the outside to the lungs and vice versa.

HOW TO INSERT AN NPA

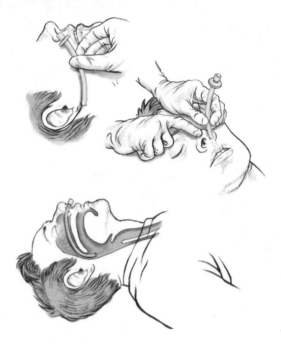

Choose the correct NPA length by holding a few sizes next to the person's face. Pick the one that goes from the bottom of the nostril to the tip of the earlobe. Apply a water-soluble lubricant to the tube.

Push the tip of the victim's nose up. Insert the NPA into a nostril with the device's beveled opening pointed toward the nose's septum (center). Push the NPA in until the flange is flush with the nostril opening. If you have trouble, try again with the other nostril.

CHOKING

If a foreign body gets caught in the throat, it can block the airway completely and make it impossible to breathe. The current thinking is, even if you suspect this has happened, don't just go blindly swiping a finger through the victim's mouth, since you're likely to push the foreign body in deeper.

THE UNIVERSAL SIGN OF CHOKING

Silently grabbing the throat with both hands is known as the universal sign of choking. Note the "silently" part. When the airway is completely blocked, no air can get by, so there's no cough or speech. If there's coughing, that may well dislodge the foreign body without any intervention.

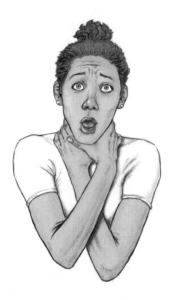

The universal sign of choking

ABDOMINAL THRUSTS

If someone is eating and suddenly goes completely silent, with a look of panic on his face, ask, "Are you choking?"

If there's a nod signaling yes, then, for legal purposes, ask, "Can I help?"

If there's another nod, perform abdominal thrusts (also sometimes called the Heimlich maneuver). Get behind the victim and put your arms around his waist. Make a fist, with the thumb side touching his abdomen, and center it just below the breastbone. Place your other hand over your fist and bend the victim slightly forward, pushing with your chest.

Now push your fist inward and upward, hard and fast. Repeat this five times. If there's no cough or sign of airflow, repeat it five more times, and again. If the airway does not become unblocked and the victim starts losing consciousness, help him to the floor. Begin chest compressions (see page 141) only after he's unconscious.

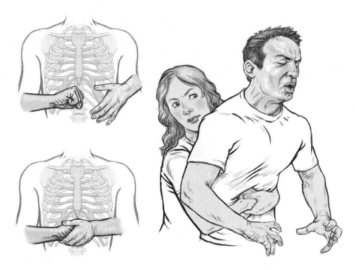

Abdominal thrusts for choking

If your arms aren't long enough to fit around the abdomen, you can try encircling and pushing on the lower chest. If you still have no luck, you may have to try to get the victim to lie down so you can push on the upper abdomen from that position.

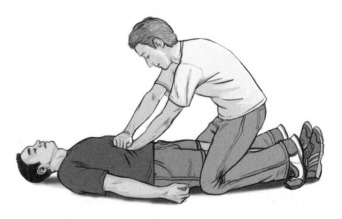

Abdominal thrusts in lying position

Abdominal Thrusts for Pregnant Women

Instead of pushing the upper abdomen, perform the thrusts on the lower chest.

Abdominal Thrusts for Babies

If a choking child stops breathing and is small enough for you to do this method with her, sit down and rest your arm on your thigh. Prop the baby facedown on your arm with her head lower than her chest. With the heel of your hand, give her five sharp hits between the shoulder blades. Then turn the baby over and perform five chest compressions (see page 141) using your index and middle fingers. If there's no response, turn the baby facedown again and repeat. If the baby loses consciousness, start two-finger chest compressions.

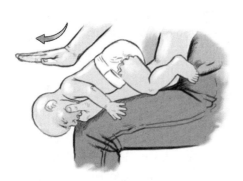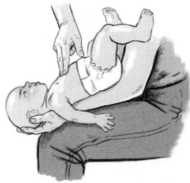

What to do for a choking baby

Agonal Breathing

When is breathing not really breathing? When it's agonal breathing. And it can fool you when you're checking for signs of life.

Even if a victim has no heartbeat—is clinically dead—the chest and diaphragm muscles may occasionally move, resulting in what seems like a quick and desperate gasp for air. But this muscle reflex is so inefficient that it carries no substantial air to the lungs. It's not really breathing and not a sign of life.

Agonal breathing is sporadic and occurs at a rate of six or fewer "breaths" per minute.

ARTIFICIAL RESPIRATION

Most adults who suddenly collapse and die were breathing just fine until their hearts stopped pumping. At the moment of collapse, they still have a pretty good level of oxygen in their blood, so the current thinking is that bystanders should concentrate on giving quality chest compressions (see page 141) to get that blood pumping again rather than adding artificial respiration.

But there are some instances when lack of adequate breathing is the most likely reason for collapse. In those cases, artificial respiration is a must. Some common examples of victims who fall in this category are:

- Prepubescent children—you can assume a child hasn't reached puberty if there is no underarm or genital hair and no breast development (the reason for collapse in this age group is more likely breathing problems, such as choking, than heart problems)

- People who have drowned

- Victims of drug overdoses

To perform artificial respiration, first make sure the airway is open by doing the jaw thrust or head tilt (see page 157). Then pinch the victim's nostrils closed and seal your mouth over his open mouth. Blow. If you don't see the chest rise, readjust the airway. Perform thirty chest compressions (see page 141) followed by two breaths. Repeat.

In small children, you can seal your mouth over the victim's nose and mouth. And be careful. The smaller the child, the less hard you have to blow. It only takes a little puff for a baby; anything stronger than that could actually injure his lungs.

To protect yourself against oral secretions, you can punch a hole in a piece of plastic or a glove and place it over the victim's mouth. Better yet, buy several disposable barriers with one-way valves and keep them in your first aid kits. These small and affordable devices allow you to blow air in, but the victim's secretions can't get out.

9

THE ABDOMEN—
NEVER SPILL
YOUR GUTS

POP QUIZ

You're in the storm of the century and start having pain in the right side of your abdomen, up along the rib-cage area—gallbladder territory. The pain comes and goes but is getting more severe. You stop eating and hope it goes away, but it only gets worse. In fact, soon your whole abdomen is hurting. Just the subtle jars from walking give you terrific pain. What's your best option?

A. Start antibiotics and continue not eating or drinking anything.

B. Drink more water, because one of your problems is dehydration.

C. Watch and wait. Give it twenty-four hours and see if it gets better.

D. Get to a medical facility if there's any way possible, even by air transport.

ANSWERS

A. Incorrect. This is your second-best option. If there's no way to get to medical facility, and you can't happen to find a doctor willing to do surgery on the kitchen table (like an MD did for my father's appendicitis in the 1920s), antibiotics will have to do.

B. Incorrect. If you've ever had abdominal surgery, you were probably told not to eat or drink anything until you pass gas. That's because if something irritates the outside of the intestine, it just shuts down and stops working. Food, liquids, and gas stay where they are and the gas keeps building. The intestine may get so bloated that it springs a leak. Then you're in real trouble (see page 168).

C. Incorrect. As hinted in answer B, this problem is a true emergency and death is common. Getting to a facility that can find the underlying cause and fix it quickly is essential. Often surgery is the only option.

D. Correct. The pain from walking gives it away. With abdominal pain, one of the big worries is that some digestive-tract contents could be leaking into the abdominal cavity, which can be a life-threatening emergency. At that point, finding out where the leak is coming from is not important. It could be a severely infected gallbladder or a ruptured appendix (appendicitis pain is sometimes felt that high in the body) or something else. The leak will cause extreme irritation and probable infection of the entire abdominal cavity. Usually touching the abdomen, walking, shaking, coughing, or anything that moves its contents even a little can cause severe pain throughout it. For your best odds of surviving, you're going to need intensive care, intravenous antibiotics, and probably surgery.

TRAUMA

Trauma to the abdomen can result from a penetrating wound or any fall, hit, or jar that causes the organs or blood vessels to indirectly bruise or tear.

PUNCTURE WOUNDS

If you get stabbed in the gut, hope the object doesn't go deep. Whether it's caused by a knife, gunshot, stick, or whatever, a puncture wound to the abdomen is treated like any other puncture wound—as long as it just involves skin, fat, and muscle. Decide whether to pull the object out (see page 169), then stop the bleeding, and clean the wound well (see page 169).

But if the wound enters the abdominal cavity, all bets are off. In that situation, the immediate, life-threatening concern is any injured and bleeding blood vessels that are too deep to apply pressure to. Next, you hope the intestines and other organs haven't been punctured and are leaking. At the very least, you know the wound has exposed the entire inner abdomen to potentially life-threatening germs from the outside.

Unless you have fancy equipment or are trained to open the abdomen up and peer inside, you just don't know what's going on in there. So what in the world can you do? Well, there are some clues that can help you estimate how dire the situation is and a few general things you might be able to do until you can get help.

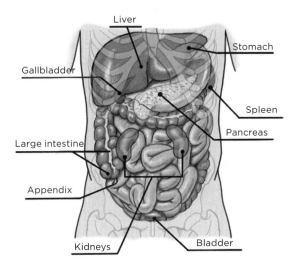

CLUES TO INTERNAL INJURY

It's not always clear how deep a wound is. Depending on the width of the wound, you might be able to see that it's entered the abdominal cavity, or you might be able to assume it has by the length of the object that's caused the injury.

You can also look for hints that something's damaged in there.

Indirect Signs of Bleeding

Signs of internal bleeding include:

- Falling blood pressure (a systolic reading of less than 90)
- A weak pulse
- A pulse rate over 100
- Dizziness
- A losing or loss of consciousness

Signs of Intestinal Leakage

Suspect that the intestines are punctured when the victim has any of these symptoms:

- Fever

- Sweating

- Tenderness not only around the wound but also over the entire abdomen

Peritoneal Signs That an Organ Is Leaking

If something in the abdomen is leaking, a clear warning is the development of peritonitis, or inflammation of the peritoneum, and it means you need to get expert help fast.

A thin membrane, called the peritoneum, lines the entire inner abdominal cavity and covers many of the organs. If it comes in contact with any chemicals or germs, like from leaking organs, then not just the area of contact but the whole lining, and hence the entire abdominal cavity, becomes inflamed.

Signs include:

- **Guarding:** The abdominal muscles spasm, and the abdominal wall becomes very tight. It's your body's way of protecting itself.

- **Rebound tenderness:** Gently press on the abdomen and let go. The letting go, or rebounding, causes severe pain. In fact, often, any movement that shakes the abdomen can cause pain.

A person with peritonitis needs expert help immediately. Lack of prompt treatment with intravenous antibiotics results in a very high risk of sepsis—an extremely serious type of infection that affects the whole body—and death. And emergency surgery may be the only way to stop the internal bleeding or leakage.

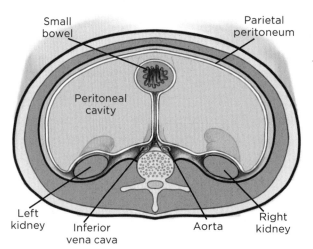

Small bowel

Parietal peritoneum

Peritoneal cavity

Left kidney

Inferior vena cava

Aorta

Right kidney

Cross section of the abdomen. The peritoneum lines the inner wall of the abdomen and covers several organs and blood vessels. The space between the linings is called the peritoneal cavity.

TREATMENT

For any signs of peritonitis or internal bleeding, immediate transfer to a medical facility is essential. If the object that you suspect punctured the abdominal cavity is still embedded, keep it in place and protect it against movement. This is to avoid further injury, and it may help the doctor home in on the area of damage. Also, if you remove the object, you may be removing the only thing stopping the bleeding or the leaking. (Of course, if expert help is unavailable for days, you'll have to make a judgment call about when to remove it.)

Here are some additional guidelines:

- If the wound is so large that some of the abdominal contents are poking out, poking them back in is likely to cause a massive infection. Just keep the area moist with a wet covering; otherwise, the exposed contents will dry out and die.

- Pack the wound to at least stop as much bleeding as you can. Tampons are often a good alternative for packing if the wound is narrow.

- Have the victim rest.

- Give the victim no food or drink as long as there are signs of peritonitis and as long as he is not passing gas. (Passing gas is a sign the intestines are moving stuff along; no gas means the contents are just sitting there.)

- Give the victim antibiotics if you have them.

- IV fluids, if you have them, should be used judiciously. Although the victim will need them to keep from getting dehydrated, giving them too fast could raise blood pressure and impede clotting.

The truth is that many stab and gunshot wounds that have penetrated the abdominal cavity don't hit vital stuff. And without expert care, tests, and possibly surgery for a direct look, it can be difficult to tell which wounds have. Many times all you may be able to do, other than try the above guidelines, is wait and hope for the best.

BLUNT TRAUMA

Anything within the abdomen can get bruised by a direct hit to the abdominal wall. Organs, blood vessels, and tissues that attach them to the abdominal wall and to each other can also be injured by a sudden stop at an accelerated speed, as you'd experience in a car wreck or a fall.

THE ABDOMEN—NEVER SPILL YOUR GUTS

Clues

The main clues that indicate bruising are pretty simple: tenderness or swelling localized to the injured area. For instance, if the right upper abdomen is tender, the liver could be bruised. If the tenderness is in the left upper abdomen, the problem could be with the spleen. A bruised kidney would be felt in the flank. And if some of the blood from the bruise seeps out into the surrounding tissue, bruising might actually be seen on the skin.

If the trauma has caused a leak in the organs, signs of peritonitis (see page 168) are likely. If the trauma has injured a blood vessel, you should see indirect clues of internal bleeding (see page 167).

Treatment

The usual treatment for internal bruising is rest and eating only small amounts of easily digestible foods. Many bruises will heal with time. Sometimes, however, bleeding can be severe, and surgery is needed to stop it.

Signs of peritonitis would be treated the same way as if a puncture wound had caused them (see page 166). And internal bleeding needs immediate expert care, if possible.

ABDOMINAL PAIN

Finding the cause of abdominal pain can be quite the challenge. In fact, it can sometimes be next to impossible without sophisticated tests or exploratory surgery.

And to make it even more complicated, every once in a while, abdominal pain isn't even caused by an abdominal problem. For example, pneumonia can start out masquerading as upper abdominal pain. So if expert help and equipment are not available, we do what we can and pay attention to the clues our body gives us.

Fortunately the abdomen does have one convenient characteristic: its squishiness. Yes, even if a victim has rock-hard abs, it's possible to press around in there and find specific areas of tenderness. This technique is called palpation. Press firmly but not hard enough to cause further injury. You can actually palpate anywhere on the body, though the abdomen is the only place where you can palpate organs because there are no bones protecting them.

I remember so well, in my first years of practice, treating the sweetest little girl who had pain in her wrist. I palpated the bones until I found the area of tenderness. She jerked her arm back and with tears in her eyes asked firmly, "Why did you *do* that?"

I felt so bad. Of course I did it to find the exact source of the pain, but how can you explain that to a five-year-old? The thing is, pain can occur far away from what's causing it, and palpating for tenderness can help you locate the actual source.

Of course, when you find the area of tenderness, you need to know which organs reside there. So for diagnostic and descriptive purposes, the abdomen is often divided into quadrants (see illustration below).

To palpate the abdomen, have the victim lie down and bend her knees slightly to relax the abdominal muscles. Feel around quadrant by quadrant. I usually start away from the place where I think the source of the pain is and press slowly and fairly gently to begin, hoping this will also help in keeping the muscles relaxed.

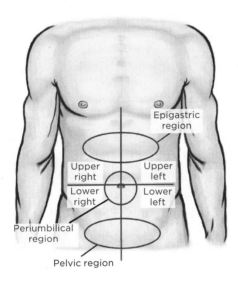

Epigastric
region

Upper
right

Upper
left

Lower
right

Lower
left

Periumbilical
region

Pelvic region

✚ HOW TO TELL A MUSCLE BRUISE FROM SOMETHING DEEPER

An injury to the muscles in the abdominal wall can cause severe pain, but, rather than needing surgery, this problem is treated like any other muscle bruise or strain. Here's a tip to determine if the pain is coming from the muscles in the abdominal wall instead of deeper:

1. Palpate the abdomen to find any localized area of tenderness— meaning a place that hurts when you press on it.

2. If you find a tender spot, have the victim tense his abdominal muscles while you're still pressing. A trick to help him tense them is to ask him to lie on his back and raise his head and shoulders, or raise both legs

without bending the knees. If the victim is a child, you could dangle your finger a couple of inches above her navel and have her try to pooch out her stomach enough to touch it. Then have her suck her stomach in and try to make it touch the spine.

3. If the tenderness from palpation persists or worsens while the muscles are contracted, and the victim won't let you press deeply due to that tenderness, it's likely coming from the muscles. If the tenderness from palpation is better when the muscles are tensed, it's likely coming from a deeper source because the tensed muscles are protecting the affected innards from your pressing.

This technique can work if the pain is fairly localized. If it's generalized, there's a risk that the pain is caused by peritonitis, because the tensing (or any abdominal movement) can make this very serious internal problem hurt worse.

RIGHT UPPER QUADRANT

The right upper quadrant of the abdomen houses the liver and gallbladder. The liver stays protected up under the rib cage. Since the bottom of the liver is concave, even the gallbladder, which is attached to it, is somewhat protected. To palpate either organ requires a little poking inward and up toward the chest. Another trick is to press just below the rib cage and have the person take a deep breath. That lowers the diaphragm and pushes part of the liver and gallbladder from the protection of the rib cage down toward your hand.

Liver

If the liver is tender, hepatitis (liver inflammation) is a likely cause. Nausea, fatigue, and fever are common symptoms. The skin and the whites of the eyes have a yellow tinge (jaundice), and the urine can be very dark.

Hepatitis can be caused by anything that inflames the liver, such as certain medicines or a flare-up of the chronic disease cirrhosis. But viruses are the most common cause. Hepatitis B and C are spread through blood and semen of someone who has the virus. Hepatitis A is spread through feces—the same way many stomach viruses are spread.

All types of hepatitis are treated with rest and trying to eat and drink to keep your body going until it can fight the infection off. Sometimes, especially with hepatitis B and C, specialized treatment is required.

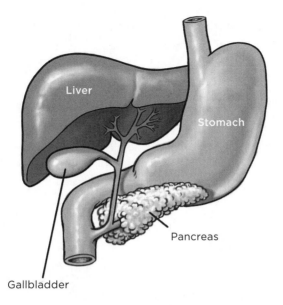

Liver

Stomach

Pancreas

Gallbladder

When Pain Goes Traveling

Sometimes, pain in one part of the body is caused by something that's not even in that area. This is called referred pain. Some of the most common examples are:

- Upper abdominal pain, which can be a symptom of pneumonia
- Pain in the lower right shoulder blade, which can be caused by gallbladder problems
- Indigestion, which can actually be a symptom of a heart attack
- Pain in the middle of the back, which could be caused by problems with the pancreas

Gallbladder

The gallbladder is a storage bag for extra bile, a digestive fluid your small intestine uses. The liver makes the bile, then it drains through a tube to the small intestine. In between, the tube branches off to the gallbladder, which will store any overflow until it's needed. Sometimes gallbladder disease causes no symptoms at all. But occasionally a sludge or stones develop in the gallbladder, either of which can inflame it and cause a low-grade ache. If one of those stones gets in the tube, the stretching of the tube's walls can cause severe pain. If the stone can't pass and the tube gets blocked, the bile backs up, causing more inflammation and sometimes infection and fever. Rarely, the gallbladder could even start leaking bile into the abdominal cavity.

Many times in an acute attack like this, severe pain comes and goes. Treatment for such a case is fasting. After a few hours, though, you'll need to take in some water, either by mouth or IV, to keep from getting dehydrated. Antibiotics may also be needed to treat infection. Of course, see a doctor if you can for a definite diagnosis and possible surgical removal of the organ. We can live without a gallbladder just fine.

EPIGASTRIC REGION

The epigastric region is the upper middle part of the abdomen. The end of stomach and the beginning of the small intestine (duodenum)—areas where many ulcers occur—as well as the pancreas reside here.

Stomach

Acid and enzymes pour into the stomach to digest food. The stomach lining is protected from these by a strong layer of mucus. Too much acid or too little mucus can lead to irritation and even an ulcer.

Stomach irritation (gastritis) and ulcers generally cause a gnawing, burning, or aching pain. In some people, the pain is relieved by eating, which probably absorbs the acid. In others, eating makes it worse. (Maybe it causes the production of more acid. We're not sure.) And sometimes certain foods—even spicy and acidic ones—help, and others don't.

If ulcers are left untreated and get worse, they may start bleeding. That causes a jet-black, tarry bowel movement. (By the way, bismuth subsalicylate, a.k.a. Pepto-Bismol, can turn your bowel movement just as black.) The bleeding may be as light as a very slight oozing or profuse. If the victim is vomiting blood, that usually means the bleeding is bad.

Sometimes the bleeding will stop on its own, but by waiting for this to happen you run a huge risk, especially if it's more than an ooze. A medical procedure done in a specialized facility may be the best way to stop it.

A perforated ulcer occurs when the ulcer eats a hole through the stomach. Stomach contents leaking through the abdominal wall causes peritonitis (see page 168), and immediate surgery to repair the leak is essential for survival.

To avoid bleeding and perforated ulcers, treat gastritis and ulcers in their early stages, when you first notice symptoms. Taking your favorite liquid or chewable antacid can help neutralize stomach acid and give short-term relief. The many prescription and over-the-counter acid blocking medicines can keep the acid from being produced. Also avoid aspirin and other anti-inflammatory medicines, alcohol, and tobacco.

But these days the cure is thought to include antibiotics because the bacterium *Helicobacter pylori* has been found to be the underlying cause of most gastritis and ulcers. More than half the world's population is infected with *H. pylori*, and it is contagious. Apparently most people live with it with no problems, but for some it causes inflammation of the stomach lining and weakens the protective mucous barrier. Since *H. pylori* has a knack for becoming resistant to antibiotics, treatment consists of a combination of several antibiotics prescribed by your health care professional.

Clues for Finding the Source of Abdominal Bleeding

Vomited blood comes from either the stomach or esophagus. It can be bright or dark red, or it can look like coffee grounds. (Gastric juices can make it black.) So if there's much bleeding in the stomach or esophagus, bowel movements will also be black.

Bleeding from the small or large intestine can color the bowel movement any color of red—but not black, unless the bleeding is very close to the connection with the stomach. Bleeding from the small intestine or the first part of the large intestine is usually maroon. Some of the many causes are infectious diarrhea, cancer, Crohn's disease, and other causes of inflammation.

Bleeding in the lower part of the large intestine or anus is usually bright red. Common causes are polyps (little protrusions in the intestinal wall), hemorrhoids, diverticula (little pockets in the intestinal wall), and cancer.

And sometimes the bleeding isn't even heavy enough to notice. A lab test to detect it may provide your only clue. Or, if the bleeding has been going on for long, another clue may be anemia.

Pancreas

Just as stomach acid can irritate the stomach, pancreatic digestive enzymes can irritate the pancreas. This problem is called pancreatitis. The two major causes are drinking too much alcohol and bile blockage from gallstones. Trauma and many medications can also cause it.

The pancreas produces digestive enzymes, along with insulin and glucagon (a hormone that raises blood sugar). A tube drains the juices into the small intestine and ends in the same opening as the tube that drains bile from the liver and gallbladder. That's why bile blockage can affect the pancreas and why pancreas problems can affect the liver.

Pancreatitis usually causes a sudden pain, like something is boring into you. The pain can get gradually worse and can radiate to the back. Other symptoms are nausea, vomiting, fever, and jaundice (yellowing of the skin and eyes from liver damage).

Allow the pancreas to rest: take in absolutely no food or liquids for a minimum of twenty-four hours or until the pain subsides, whichever is longer. IV fluids are very important during this time, not only because you're not drinking but also because the inflamed pancreas can leak a lot of fluid into the abdominal cavity. Once the pain subsides, start eating a low-fat, nondairy diet (fat and dairy products may trigger the production of more pancreatic enzymes than other food types).

If the pain doesn't subside in a day or two and you can get to a health care provider by then, having a nasogastric tube (a flexible, hollow tube that goes from the nose to the stomach) inserted and digestive juices drawn out may help.

Surgical removal of gallstones may be necessary. Antibiotics are sometimes needed, but not usually. The fever that invariably occurs with pancreatitis is usually a reaction to the inflammation and not a sign of infection. Only in severe cases, in which part of the pancreas has actually died, does infection become a problem. So given the risks of antibiotics, not to mention the probable shortage in dire situations, perhaps save them for severe cases—when the symptoms are getting worse instead of better or there are other worrisome signs, such as increasing lethargy or falling blood pressure.

But just because antibiotics may not help doesn't mean pancreatitis is not serious. Even outside of survival situations, about 10 percent of people with pancreatitis die because of complications or the failure of other organs.

DOCTOR SPEAK

When referring to disease, the suffix "itis" means inflammation. Inflammation is a reaction to something that irritates, and it can cause such things as redness, warmth, swelling, pain, and tenderness. Infection (from a bacteria, virus, fungus, or parasite) is one cause of irritation.

LEFT UPPER QUADRANT

Most of the stomach resides in the left upper quadrant of the abdomen. The spleen does, too. Like the liver on the right side, the spleen is protected by the rib cage. So palpate the spleen using the same techniques: do a little poking, or press under the rib cage and have the person take a deep breath.

Stomach

Excess gas can stretch the stomach, causing pain and tenderness. But most ulcer and gastritis pain is more in the epigastric area, where the stomach ends and empties into the small intestine. (This is where the right and left upper quadrants intersect).

Spleen

The spleen is part of your immune system. It screens out bacteria. Think of it as a really big lymph node with a really good blood supply. It also catches and gets rid of old, damaged red blood cells to make room in the bloodstream for new ones.

The main concern regarding the spleen is injury. This is usually the cause of significant tenderness, and a direct hit to the spleen can cause a blood leak or worse. If there's a large leak or a rupture, there may be widespread abdominal pain plus indirect signs of blood loss, such as a drop in blood pressure or a fast pulse.

If the leak is small, sometimes the bleeding stops on its own. Occasionally, the spleen can rupture, resulting in massive blood loss and requiring emergency surgery to stop the bleeding. You can live without a spleen, but you will be more susceptible to certain infections.

RIGHT LOWER QUADRANT

The appendix is little wormlike pouch coming off the large intestine close to where it connects with the small intestine. It usually resides in the right lower quadrant of the abdomen. We're not sure what useful function it might have, but it certainly appears that we have no problem living without one. In women, the right ovary (see page 197) and fallopian tube (see page 196) are also located in this vicinity, sometimes making it difficult to discern if the ovary, fallopian tube, or appendix is the cause of pain and tenderness.

Appendicitis occurs if hardened feces or mucus blocks the appendix opening. Bacteria build up, and the appendix gets infected. The condition often starts with a vague pain in the midabdomen. With time it localizes in the right lower quadrant and becomes more severe. But pain from the appendix is notorious for occasionally showing up as tenderness in just about any part of the abdomen. Nausea and lack of appetite are common but don't always occur. If the appendix ruptures, it will usually cause peritonitis, with all the symptoms and dangers that go with it.

Treatment is surgery to remove the appendix. If that's impossible, there is a chance that antibiotics and time will help a mild case heal. Or, even if the appendix ruptures, the infection may wall off into an abscess whether you're taking antibiotics or not. The abscess may at least temporarily keep the infection from draining into the abdomen and causing peritonitis. But as a rule, it's best to not take chances. In most cases, if we suspect an appendix is inflamed, it is surgically removed.

LEFT LOWER QUADRANT

The small and large intestines extend across all four quadrants of the abdomen, but the lowest section of the large intestine, before it empties into the rectum, resides here, and this section is where common intestinal problems most often occur. In women, the left ovary (see page 197) and fallopian tube (see page 196) are located here also.

Sometimes the large intestine develops little pockets or pouches (kind of like the appendix) called diverticula. If you have these pouches, you have diverticulosis, which only means the pockets are there. It's more of a condition than a disease. Many people have them and never know it unless tests are done or unless one of them gets stopped up, inflamed, and infected. That problem is called diverticulitis. It just so happens that the part of the large intestine that resides in the left lower quadrant is where the most diverticula occur. Along with pain and tenderness in the area, diverticulitis may cause fever.

Treatment is antibiotics. Unlike appendicitis, diverticulitis rarely requires surgical removal of the infected pocket. Also rarely, an infected diverticulum can leak, causing the dreaded peritonitis.

Nothing prevents the formation of diverticula. And nothing has been shown to prevent diverticulitis. But eating a lot of fiber is generally recommended for the latter. This bulks up your bowel movements and puts less pressure on the insides of your intestines, potentially making bouts of inflammation less likely. Some experts have recommended not eating seeds and nuts if you have diverticulosis, but recent studies have shown no risk from those foods. Still, I know some patients and doctors who would say from firsthand experience that seeds and nuts can cause a problem in some people.

Tips for a Relaxed Abdominal Exam

It seems like every child I've ever treated for abdominal pain has pointed to his or her belly button when I've asked where it hurts. When you're palpating a child's abdomen, the key is to get his mind on something else while casually pressing around. Watch his expression carefully. Start fairly lightly. If there's no reaction, press a little harder. He'll wince or let you know in other ways if a particular spot is tender. In fact, depending on the amount of pain, one press in a tender spot may be all you get. If there's no tenderness anywhere, there's a good chance that the pain may not be caused by a problem that needs surgery.

Many adults, also, automatically tense their abdominal muscles during an exam. Talking about something else can help them relax. When they're lying down (which they should be for an abdominal exam), having them bend their knees also helps relax the abdominal muscles.

Another option for children is take the child's hand in yours and allow her to touch her own abdomen, with your hand on top providing pressure. If that doesn't work, having her sit in a parent's lap can make her relax enough for you to work in some semblance of an exam.

For a crying baby, a pacifier may help.

MIDLOWER ABDOMEN (PELVIS)

The midlower abdomen holds the bladder and the uterus. For uterus problems see page 192.

On any given late Friday afternoon, I'm never surprised to see a woman or three show up, asking to be worked in before the clinic closes. And I can pretty well guess their problem. They've started having a little burning when urinating, or they feel like they have to go to the bathroom all the time. They've had the problem before and know how intense the symptoms can get, and they don't want to suffer through the weekend or go the emergency room for something that seems so minor but hurts so badly.

It's estimated that between 20 and 50 percent of women—as opposed to only about 1 or 2 percent of men—will have at least one bladder infection in their lifetimes. When you have a bladder infection, the urine itself often appears normal, but it's not unusual for it to have a cloudy appearance and an odor. And sometimes the bladder wall gets so irritated that the urine becomes bloody.

Even if the urine is bloody, taking antibiotics—such as sulfa drugs, floxins, or even amoxicillin—for a few days and drinking plenty of water should clear up the problem. There are also over-the-counter medicines that ease the burning and the feeling of urgency. Sitting in a warm tub of water for fifteen or twenty minutes can help soothe these symptoms, too.

Eating cranberries or drinking unsweetened cranberry juice can keep bacteria from sticking to the bladder wall. It's still unclear whether this actually treats or prevents an infection, but in any case, consume only moderate amounts, because too much can cause stomach upset and diarrhea.

To help prevent urinary tract infections, adopt these habits:

• Drink lots of water and other fluids to flush things out.

• Limit caffeine, since it can irritate the bladder.

• Don't hold urine for long periods of time, since the longer the urine pools in the bladder, the more time bacteria have to multiply in it.

• Urinate immediately after sex to clear out any bacteria near the urethra.

• Wear cotton underwear and breathable fabrics, and don't stay in wet clothes any longer than you must, since bacteria love moisture.

• Avoid harsh soap, douches, and any chemicals that could irritate the surrounding area.

DOCTOR SPEAK

A urinary tract infection is an infection occurring anywhere along the urinary tract, from the urethra to the kidney.

Urethritis is infection of the urethra (the tube that empties the bladder). Cystitis is infection or inflammation of the bladder. Pyelonephritis is infection of the kidney. That's the dangerous one—it can cause fever and infection in the bloodstream and may require hospitalization (see page 182). In reality, though, most people refer to just about any of these conditions simply as a kidney infection. It's your health care worker's job to discern the specifics.

General Advice for Abdominal Pain

If you think your abdominal pain is from a kidney or bladder infection, drink lots of fluids. Otherwise, don't eat or drink for at least for a few hours. If your abdomen hurts all over, don't eat or drink at all until the pain subsides. In that case, you may need IV fluids to keep from getting dehydrated.

These are general guidelines until you can get checked. There are always exceptions.

SIDE OR BACK OF THE ABDOMEN

The kidneys reside on each side of the abdomen, just above the hip bones. So problems with the kidneys can cause pain in the side or the back. But a less obvious potential cause of back pain is an abdominal aortic aneurysm.

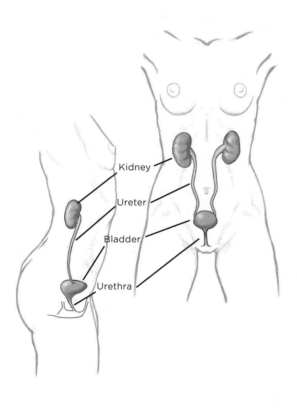

Kidney

Ureter

Bladder

Urethra

The Kidneys

The two most common kidney problems are infection and kidney stones. Infection causes tenderness in the area; kidney stones don't. Instead, they may cause severe pain, usually around the kidney area and radiating into the groin.

One way to check the kidney is to push that soft spot in the back between the lower ribs and hip. The area will be tender if the kidney is inflamed.

A kidney infection, called pyelonephritis, is an infection that's gone beyond the bladder and into the kidney. Treatment is generally the same as for a bladder infection. Vomiting or fever over 101 is a sign that the infection is getting into the bloodstream and that the victim may need IV antibiotics.

Kidney stones may stay up in the actual kidney without pain. But if one gets into the ureter—the tube that drains urine from the kidney into the bladder—the pain can be severe when it tries to push the stone along. In between pushes, there's no pain.

With time, either the stone will pass into the bladder or it will get stuck in the tube, potentially causing a blockage that can severely damage the kidney. Either way, the pain may stop for good, but if it's stuck it may be causing permanent damage.

So at the first sign of a kidney stone, drink lots of fluids, in the hope that they will push the stone to the bladder. Take pain medicine if you have it. Walking may make the stone move. When passing kidney stones, it really is true: no pain, no gain.

If a stone does get stuck and doesn't start moving within a few days, it will need to be removed by a doctor, so it's important to know if you've urinated it out. Many times the stone is so small you won't notice it. In that case, unless you have special testing, you may not know the reason the pain has stopped: is it because the stone is stuck and not moving, or is it because you've actually passed it? One solution is to urinate into a coffee filter or some other strainer during your attack so you'll catch most anything that comes through. Sometimes the stone can be so small you'll be amazed it could have caused so much pain.

The Aorta

The aorta is the large artery that connects to your heart. As with any artery, it's possible for the wall to become weak in one spot and balloon out. That's called an aortic aneurysm. One clue that you have this problem can be a pulsating or throbbing around your navel. Another clue is a constant back pain or deep abdominal pain. But many times there are no symptoms.

If the aorta leaks or tears, it may cause a severe, searing pain in the abdomen or back and pain down both legs. You may also have a drop in blood pressure, a fast pulse, and even loss of consciousness. Immediate surgery is often lifesaving. Otherwise, there is no treatment except to rest and hope for the best. On the other hand, if your blood pressure is extremely high instead of low and you have some blood pressure medicine, taking it might help ease the pressure on the aortic wall.

The Abdominal Lymph Nodes

The abdomen has lymph nodes. Just like with other lymph nodes, many viral and bacterial infections cause them to be tender, even infections not in the abdomen. The pain is usually not severe. There's no specific treatment, and the pain will go away when the infection does.

HERNIA

When I'm doing routine physicals on men, I save the hernia check for last. Here's how it goes.

"Okay, now I need to check you for a hernia," I announce as I'm snapping on a glove.

Big sigh. "Oh, Doc."

If the patient's wife is in the room, she smiles, stands up, and says, "I'll wait outside." Sometimes I hear a "Your turn," as she shuts the door.

It's now me and the guy. I sit on a stool.

"Okay," I say. "Please face me and pull your pants down. Underwear, too."

The guy fumbles around like his belt and zipper aren't working. "Doc, I've always wondered. What exactly is a hernia?"

I never know if he's really curious or just stalling for time. Anyway, here's the scoop. And, by the way, women get hernias, too.

A hernia is a weak spot or tear that allows contents, which are usually held in, to protrude out. With an abdominal hernia, part of the small intestine protrudes through a weak spot or tear in an abdominal muscle. This causes a soft, usually nontender bulge that gets larger with standing up and straining and goes away when you're lying down.

Common types of abdominal hernias are:

- **Inguinal:** In men, the inguinal canal is where the spermatic cord travels into the scrotum. In women, a ligament resides there that helps hold up the uterus. Inguinal hernias occur mostly in men.

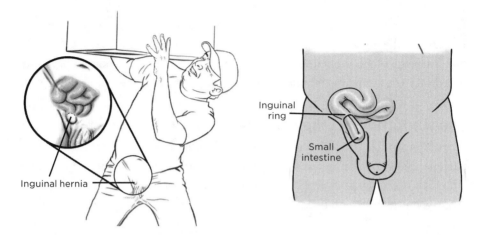

The drawing on the left illustrates the inguinal canal starting to weaken or tear. In the drawing on the right, the hernia has progressed, and the intestine is poking through.

- **Femoral:** In the groin, there's a little channel where the femoral artery travels from the abdomen down into the thigh, and that's where a femoral hernia may occur.

- **Umbilical:** Your navel is the scar that's left where your umbilical cord used to be. Some people are born with a weak spot there, or muscle weakness can develop with age. Obesity is a risk factor.

- **Incisional:** A hernia can happen where a surgical wound didn't heal completely.

Turn Your Head and Cough

Other than "Turn around and bend over," "Turn your head and cough" are the words men dread the most during a routine physical. So what exactly are we doctors checking? We're poking our fingers up into the inguinal canal. The cough produces abdominal pressure, so if there's a tear or a weak spot, the intestine will poke out. Any straining would produce the same result. Coughing is just the standard way to check. And the "Turn your head" part? That's so you don't cough on the doctor.

CAUSES

Some people are born with weakness in the inguinal, femoral, or umbilical region. That alone can cause a hernia, or that plus persistent straining (like from heavy lifting), a chronic cough, and even constipation. Obesity and smoking can also weaken the muscles. Occasionally, an otherwise normal muscle may tear from trauma.

TREATMENT

Stop straining. It can make the hernia grow larger. A restrictive undergarment called a truss might make you feel better, but it won't do anything to actually treat the hernia. And it can give you a false sense of security.

Surgery to repair the weak or torn spot is the only definitive treatment. It can also help avoid the rare but sometimes fatal complications incarceration and strangulation. They have nothing to do with crime, but they are scary—and deadly serious.

Incarceration happens when part of the small intestine gets caught in the hernia and can't get back out. This kinks the intestine so that feces and even gas can't move and be expelled. The area swells, making the trapped piece of intestine even more constricted. There can be tremendous pain.

If the trapped piece is not released, the swelling will eventually cut off circulation to that part of the intestine. That's called strangulation. When that happens, unless surgery is performed within hours, that part of the intestine will die and become gangrenous, which makes the victim even sicker. Without surgery at that point, death will ensue.

ACUTE INFECTIOUS DIARRHEA

"Infectious" is the key word here. I'm not talking about the diarrhea that's often one of many symptoms of a chronic disease; nor am I talking about food intolerances. Rather, I'm talking about stomach viruses, food poisoning, and the stomach flu (not really the flu, but it is a virus). I'm also talking about diarrhea caused by bacteria and parasites, in which germs either directly cause inflammation of the intestinal lining or produce a toxin that does the dirty work for them. In time, the germs are expelled and the symptoms go away, although sometimes antibiotics are needed if a bacterial infection is severe.

CLUES

Besides frequent watery bowel movements, symptoms may include vomiting, fever, aches and pains, weakness, gas, bloating, and abdominal pain.

TREATMENT

Supplements that have been shown to shorten the course of diarrhea are probiotics (healthful live bacteria and yeasts)—such as *lactobacilli, bifidobacteria,* and *Saccharomyces boulardii*—and zinc.

Diarrhea's therapeutic mainstay—and often the only treatment needed until the diarrhea runs its course—is dehydration prevention, because diarrhea can take a lot of fluid out of your body. Water is the immediate need, but if the diarrhea is profuse or prolonged, the loss of sodium and potassium can become significant. And at some point, your body will need calories.

Eating salted crackers could help, too, if you can tolerate them. Pedialyte and Gastrolyte may balance the body's fluids and electrolytes without aggravating the diarrhea. Broth, watered-down sports drinks, or watered-down fruit juices will also usually do the trick.

Start with small sips. If there's vomiting, wait a few hours and try again. If you still vomit up the fluids, wait a few more hours. Vomiting from infectious diarrhea is usually gone within twenty-four hours, but IV fluids, if available, can help prevent dehydration. The IV may be required earlier in small children, elderly people, and people with chronic diseases.

Breast-feeding should continue, whether it's the baby with the problem, the mother, or both, although if the mother's the sick one, she'll need to ingest more fluids than if she weren't nursing.

Because getting commercial fluids such as Pedialyte and Gastrolyte, which contain just the right amount of electrolytes and carbohydrates, may be impossible for some people, the World Health Organization offers an oral rehydration salts packet that can be dissolved in clean water. The WHO says the packets can treat up to 80 percent of even the worst cases of diarrhea if they're used properly. The packets are fairly cheap and easy to store.

If you don't have these packets, you can make your own rehydration salts using the recipe on page 187, but be sure to measure ingredients accurately. Too much sugar will make the diarrhea worse. Too much salt could be dangerous. Use a measuring device if you can.

After the diarrhea has settled down, you can try some solid food, but start small. It used to be standard procedure to follow the BRAT diet—bananas, rice, applesauce, and toast—but that's gone out of favor because the diet doesn't have enough protein and the foods are no better tolerated than other foods. Still, trial and error may be needed. People tend to have trouble tolerating milk for a few days after diarrhea subsides. Also, greasy or spicy foods may be hard to digest.

Recipe for Homemade Rehydration Salts

MEASURE INGREDIENTS EXACTLY.

- 1 quart or 1 liter drinkable water

- 6 level teaspoons sugar or 10 teaspoons (50 ml) honey

- 1/2 level teaspoon salt

This version lacks potassium. To add that, you can have a bite of banana or add one of the following ingredients to the above mixture:

- 1/2 cup (4 ounces) orange juice

- 1/4 level teaspoon salt substitute made of potassium, such as NoSalt

Mix well. According to the World Health Organization, people with diarrhea should drink the following amounts to avoid dehydration:

Children less than two years old: 1/4–1/2 cup (50–100 ml, or 2–3 ounces) after each loose stool; up to 1/2 quart (or 1/2 liter) per day

Children two to nine years old: 1/2–1 cup (100–200 ml, or 3–7 ounces) after each loose stool; up to 1 quart (or 1 liter) per day

People ten years old and older: As much as they want, up to 2 quarts per day

If the sick person seems to be getting dehydrated, give 1 to 1.5 ounces per pound of body weight (60–100 ml per kilogram) within a four-hour period in small sips.

What About Vomiting?

Like diarrhea, vomiting can easily cause dehydration. Staying hydrated is trickier in this case, though, because drinking fluids may trigger more vomiting—and therefore the loss of even more electrolytes. But if the person doesn't drink at all, dehydration is bound to result.

So first, have the person try just sipping fluids—the same ones that are good for diarrhea (see page 186)—to see if they stay down. If they don't, I recommend waiting about 30 minutes to an hour before trying again. The goal is to eventually work up to the recommended amount of fluids per day (see page 187).

SIGNS OF DEHYDRATION

In many countries, dehydration is the most common cause of death from acute infectious diarrhea. The following are some signs of dehydration. If you see them, give the victim even more fluids if she can keep them down, or get expert help if possible:

- **Dizziness upon standing**

- **Tenting of the skin:** Normally, if you pinch skin, it goes right back down where it came from after you let go. But if you pinch dehydrated skin, it stays up, like a tent that's been raised. However, heed the sign cautiously: the skin of elderly people who are not dehydrated may tent even when they're not dehydrated.

- **Dry tongue**

- **Decreased urination**

- **Dark yellow urine:** A general way to watch for dehydration is to note the urine color at the beginning of the illness. If, in time, it starts noticeably getting darker, that can be an early sign of dehydration.

In a small child, look for sunken eyes, a dry tongue, or few or no tears when crying. A decrease in wet diapers is also a sign, but it might be hard to notice when a child has diarrhea.

TIPS FOR WHETHER TO GIVE ANTIBIOTICS

Since antibiotics can make symptoms worse even when bacteria are causing the diarrhea, they're used sparingly. Without access to lab tests for a diagnosis, it can be a guessing game as to whether any particular bout of diarrhea is the kind antibiotics would be good for.

Traveler's diarrhea is often treated with ciprofloxacin or azithromycin. Other clues that might steer you toward antibiotics would be a high fever and blood mixed in the stool. (If the blood appears only on the toilet paper, it's usually from anal irritation caused by the diarrhea—or a hemorrhoid flaring up—and not a sign of infection.)

Another infection that causes diarrhea and can linger if not killed with antiparasitic medicine is giardia. You can get this from drinking lake or stream water that hasn't been adequately disinfected. Although you can get many other diarrhea-causing bacteria and viruses this way, too, if the diarrhea lingers for days, giardia could be the cause and metronidazole, an antiparasitic/antibiotic, the cure.

POISONING

If you suspect that someone has taken an overdose of medicine or ingested a poison, read any available label information, and immediately call the national poison control centers help line at 1-800-222-1222. Keep the number handy on your wall, in your cell phone, and on your speed dial.

Unless specifically instructed to do so, never induce vomiting. Current research suggests it doesn't help. Syrup of ipecac, the classic vomit-inducing remedy, is no longer recommended. Studies have not shown that it works, and vomiting increases the risk of esophageal damage and accidental aspiration—in other words, you could choke on your own vomit.

If expert consultation and care are impossible to get, and if activated charcoal is available, it's relatively safe and worth a try. Now, this is not the charcoal used on a grill. Rather, it's a fine granular charcoal (carbon) that has been treated to develop an enormous number of microscopic holes and to have an electrostatic attraction to certain chemical molecules. It can be bought over the counter as granules, capsules, and various other forms. It's usually kept in the dietary-supplement or health-food section. It's also an ingredient in many aquarium filters.

If used, activated charcoal should be given within an hour of the poisoning and only if the victim is fully alert and cooperative. Activated charcoal is pretty good at getting many types of medications to stick to it and does the same for some toxins but not others. For instance, giving activated charcoal is not recommended if petroleum products or household acidic or alkaline liquids are involved.

The dosage is about 0.5 gram per kilogram of body weight or 0.3 gram per pound of body weight. (A teaspoon of activated charcoal weighs about four to seven grams.) If the activated charcoal is in granule form, mix it thoroughly with water. Never mix it with foods or sweeteners that aren't already in the charcoal product, since that may cause it not to work.

Activated charcoal can cause constipation. For that reason, some brands will premix it with sorbitol. However, this mixture may cause profuse diarrhea in some.

10

FOR WOMEN ONLY

POP QUIZ

The middle-aged woman dressed in business attire sitting on the exam table states that she's had a very smelly vaginal discharge for more than a week. No fever, no pain, just the discharge. She's never had anything like this, and it's made her start wondering if her husband has been unfaithful.

When I do a pelvic exam, in the very back of her vagina I find a wadded-up tampon. Which of the following statements are *not* true?

A. Voilà: case closed.

B. Some inserted tampons remain undetected for months.

C. An undetected tampon could cause a serious infection.

D. Undetected tampons are rare in well-groomed, nonobese women.

E. Sometimes a woman can't remember removing a tampon, but
it's not inside her.

ANSWERS

A. False. Removing the tampon will probably solve the problem, but that doesn't rule out another cause of such a discharge: sexually transmitted diseases. A test for gonorrhea and chlamydia would be prudent.

B. True. There may be no symptoms at all.

C. True. It's not usually the case, but a tampon or other foreign body can cause a serious bacterial infection and, rarely, life-threatening toxic shock syndrome.

D. False. This problem could happen to any woman who uses tampons. Grooming and size have little or no relevance here.

E. True. I've had several patients who are convinced they've forgotten to remove a tampon, but upon examination, there's nothing there.

So here's what usually happens: the tampon gets compressed until it's really small and becomes lodged way in the back of the vagina, next to the cervix. And it stays there. That's because except during childbirth, the cervix opening is way too small to allow a tampon to get through and up inside the uterus.

But a tampon can certainly be hard to detect. Looking through a speculum helps, but it's often possible to find it by feeling with a couple of fingers. Just be sure you're really thorough: feel all the way to the back wall of the vagina and encircle the cervix. If you don't find anything, well, it just might not be there. Still, always see a health care provider, if possible, if you have any new vaginal discomfort or discharge.

ISSUES WITH THE UTERUS

In a woman who's not pregnant, the uterus, a.k.a. the womb, is about one and a half inches wide and three inches long—not much larger than a big toe. The opening to

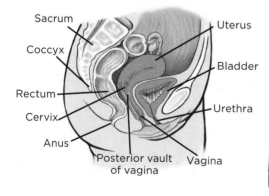

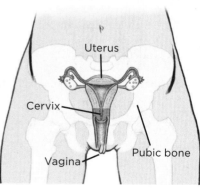

the uterus, called the cervix, connects it to the vagina and actually protrudes into the vaginal cavity a bit. It can be felt as a kind of knob in the vagina near the back. In general, a clue that there may be something wrong with the uterus is pelvic pain or bleeding.

FIBROIDS

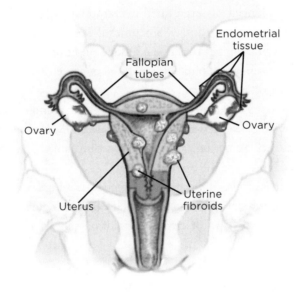

Uterine fibroids can form in various sizes and locations.

A uterine fibroid is a ball of muscle tissue within the uterine wall or attached to it. It may be miniscule or up to several inches in diameter. A majority of women will have one or more fibroids during their lifetimes. Most fibroids will never cause symptoms. The large ones are more likely to cause problems.

Fibroids can cause heavy menstrual periods and a feeling of pelvic pressure. A bimanual exam may reveal an enlarged uterus, a sign that fibroids are present. Non-steroidal anti-inflammatories (NSAIDs) may help (see page 196). Surgery or laser treatment to remove the fibroids may be required if the symptoms are really bad.

By the way, fibroids are not cancerous. Yes, they are sometimes called fibroid tumors, but it's a misconception that a tumor is a type of cancer. A tumor is just a mass of tissue. Although some tumors are cancerous, plenty of them are perfectly benign. Fibroids are benign and very rarely turn into cancers.

MISCARRIAGE

Using birth control, no matter the form, does not rule out the possibility of pregnancy. If you're a fertile female and having sexual intercourse with a man who has healthy sperm, pregnancy is always possible. Many women don't realize this, and in the early stages of pregnancy, especially if they're using birth control, they're unaware that they're expecting. It's only when they miss a menstrual period and experience the symptoms—such as breast swelling or tenderness and nausea, especially early in the morning—that they realize they're pregnant.

During pregnancy, uterine cramping and even vaginal spotting can be normal. However, prolonged or severe uterine cramping or bleeding could indicate a miscarriage or ectopic pregnancy. Sometimes if the pregnancy is early, the only clue that you're even pregnant could be a sudden onset of vaginal bleeding from a miscarriage. The discharge of pink fetal material or sometimes even a recognizable fetus could confirm the suspicion.

Often the contents of the uterus take a few weeks to completely expel, if they're going to. Continued bleeding is a clue that they haven't. Medications can help expel the remaining tissues. Sometimes a surgical procedure called dilation and curettage (D&C) is needed to scrape the uterine wall.

After a miscarriage, the uterus can get infected, causing fever, more abdominal pain, and possible vaginal discharge, in which case antibiotics are required along with complete removal of the infected material if possible.

What Is a Bimanual Exam?

An enlarged uterus, enlarged ovary, or a mass can be felt by inserting a finger or two in the vagina and pushing up on the cervix while the other hand is pressing on the midlower abdomen next to the pelvic bone. This is called a medical "bimanual" exam and can help determine the size of the uterus or any abnormal masses. If the uterus is not enlarged, the normal uterus is often too small to feel unless the woman is very thin.

PELVIC INFLAMMATORY DISEASE (PID)

Uterine infections are usually bacterial and often caused by a sexually transmitted disease that's migrated into the uterus from the vagina. Most infections of the uterus also involve the fallopian tubes (see page 196) and are lumped into the diagnosis of pelvic inflammatory disease, or PID. Scarring of the fallopian tubes can result, which can make it difficult if not impossible to get pregnant, because the egg can't get through the tubes to the uterus. Early treatment with antibiotics reduces the risk of scarring. Delaying treatment makes it more likely that the infection will get worse.

PID can cause fever, chills, and fatigue. The pain can be severe, and the infection may move into the bloodstream, where it becomes sepsis—a life-threatening, body-wide infection. On a bimanual exam, health care providers often note the "chandelier sign": just a light touch to the cervix can cause pain so severe that a patient lying on the table may jump up, hands in the air, as if she were going to grab a chandelier (or punch the examiner, I'll wager, if she had a chance).

Many times oral antibiotics will get rid of PID, but severe cases may require intravenous antibiotics. Other treatment is the same as for most infections: rest, fluids, and maybe something like an NSAID for pain.

Complications include pelvic abscesses, peritonitis (see page 168), and death. They're much less common when antibiotics are started early.

ENDOMETRIOSIS

The same type of tissue that lines the uterus—the endometrium—can sometimes grow in other parts of the pelvis, such as on the outer walls of the intestine, bladder, ovaries, and other organs. There, it responds to hormone changes just as it does in the uterus lining. During a menstrual period, it may even bleed into the pelvic cavity.

Endometriosis can cause heavy, painful periods, painful intercourse, and pain with bowel movements or urination. The same treatments that relieve menstrual cramps can help with endometriosis pain. Prescription medicines can also be used to relieve symptoms if over-the-counter remedies are not effective. Surgical removal of the tissue may be needed if symptoms are still severe.

MENSTRUAL CRAMPS

During a menstrual period, muscles in the uterus contract to expel blood. In some women these contractions can become quite painful. Two of the most commonly used remedies are NSAIDs and heat. Taking birth control pills regularly can also reduce the symptoms, as can exercising before the period and cramping start. Caffeine, smoking, and alcohol may make symptoms worse.

Some women find that regularly taking a dietary supplement helps relieve the pain. Except for the anti-inflammatory properties found in some, exactly why they help is unclear. Here are some commonly used ones:

- Fish oil (or fish) containing a lot of omega-3 fatty acids
- Vitamins B$_1$ (thiamine) and B$_6$
- Magnesium
- Fennel

- Evening primrose oil
- Vitamin D
- Calcium
- Pycnogenol

Why NSAIDs Can Ease Uterus Pain and Even Bleeding

NSAID is an abbreviation for "nonsteroidal anti-inflammatory drug." You know these drugs as ibuprofen (Advil, Motrin), naproxen (Aleve, Anaprox, Naprosyn), and many other names. They fight pain and inflammation. One way they do that is by inhibiting the body's production of the group of chemicals called prostaglandins. And it just so happens that prostaglandins are what cause muscle cramping in the uterus. Prostaglandins also increase blood flow and make platelets less sticky. So for menstrual cramps, endometriosis, and even some types of uterine bleeding, NSAIDs, by inhibiting prostaglandins, get the to source of the problem.

ISSUES WITH THE FALLOPIAN TUBES

Fallopian tubes run out from both sides of the uterus. The end of each tube flares out and covers part of the nearby ovary. So the tubes are in very close contact with the ovaries, though not attached to them. When a woman is ovulating, an egg travels the very short distance from the ovary into the fallopian tube.

ECTOPIC OR TUBAL PREGNANCY

When the egg gets fertilized by sperm, it usually happens in the fallopian tube. Then the fertilized egg keeps traveling until it attaches to the uterine wall. But if the egg gets stuck or slowed down and the pregnancy develops in the tube (a tubal pregnancy), the egg has no chance of survival. Sometimes this results in a miscarriage. But other times, severe and life-threatening bleeding can occur. If the embryo continues to grow, the fallopian tube will burst, resulting in severe peritonitis.

Rarely, the egg may get fertilized and start developing on the ovary or even in the abdominal cavity, which is called an ectopic pregnancy (actually any pregnancy outside the uterus can be called ectopic).

With an ectopic or tubal pregnancy, you will have a positive pregnancy test. You may have symptoms of pregnancy, but often, sudden pain starting on one side of the pelvis is your first clue that something is wrong. If the area starts bleeding or if the fallopian tube bursts, the pain may involve the whole pelvis.

An ultrasound can usually make a definitive diagnosis and pinpoint the location of the pregnancy. Since there is a high likelihood of unpredictable, life-threatening bleeding, immediate surgery to remove the egg or fetus and, usually, the affected part of the fallopian tube is often the treatment of choice. There are also various procedures and medications that might help the egg to pass if it's located in the tube. Sometimes the egg or fetus will just detach and pass through the tube and uterus and out the vagina on its own.

ISSUES WITH THE OVARIES

Each ovary is about the size of an almond and contains thousands of immature eggs. During a woman's fertile years, a mature egg is released once a month, on average, and enters a fallopian tube. The ovaries also produce estrogen and progesterone.

CYSTS

Sometimes a mature egg is not released and stays stuck on the ovary. Other times the egg is released but the little opening it comes through on the surface of the ovary doesn't seal properly. Either occurrence can result in a fluid-filled cyst, which is usually small, never noticed, and goes away in few months. But occasionally these cysts can grow and start causing pressure or pain. Sometimes a mass can be felt on a bimanual pelvic exam. If a big cyst bursts, the leaked fluid can cause severe pain.

Many people require no treatment. Either the cyst eventually goes away or, even if it ruptures, the pain resolves as the body absorbs the fluid. The problem, though, is that without a test such as an ultrasound, there's no definitive way to tell a benign cyst from something like an ectopic pregnancy, an abscess, or even appendicitis.

Less definitive clues that it's a cyst could be the absence of fever and other signs of infection— such as muscle aches—and a negative pregnancy test.

OVARIAN TORSION

Like every other part of your body, each ovary has a blood supply. If the main vessels going to it get twisted, the supply can be cut off—a condition called torsion— and the ovary will eventually die, resulting in a bad infection. This could in turn cause gangrene and potentially fatal peritonitis.

Ovarian torsion causes pain in the side—usually sudden, but not always—often with vomiting. There may be tenderness on that side, but sometimes it's mild, and sometimes there's no tenderness. About 20 percent of torsions occur during a pregnancy.

The treatment is surgery: nothing else will do. Occasionally the ovary can be saved, but usually it's removed.

ISSUES WITH THE VAGINA

A certain amount of vaginal discharge is normal, and each woman will know what's usual for her. Abnormal vaginal discharge can be caused by a foreign body, such as an impacted tampon (see page 192). But infection is a more common cause. Except in yeast infections, the type of discharge can't tell you exactly what the problem is without a culture or look under a microscope. But the color and odor of the discharge can sometimes provide a clue.

BACTERIAL VAGINOSIS

Bacterial vaginosis causes a thin, grayish-white discharge with a fishy smell. This comes from an imbalance in normal bacteria. Sometimes there's a slight itching on the outside of the vagina. We don't know why this happens, but risk factors include smoking and frequent douching. Bacterial vaginosis is not sexually transmitted; however, having multiple sexual partners is also a risk factor. Again, we're not sure why. Treatment is the antibiotic metronidazole, but the symptoms often recur. A tea-tree-oil douche (see page 199) might help, as could some probiotics, but the results of studies on these treatments have been pretty disappointing.

The main reason to learn to recognize bacterial vaginosis is to differentiate it from sexually transmitted diseases. The only known complications are a possible risk of early labor during pregnancy and increased susceptibility to contracting a sexually transmitted disease. Why? We don't know that either.

YEAST INFECTION

Yeast infections often cause a cottage-cheese-like, odorless discharge that attaches to the walls of the vagina. There can also be a lot of external irritation, redness, and swelling. The itching can be severe.

Because yeast is a normal component of the vagina, and because it lives on various parts of the bodies of both sexes, a yeast infection is not considered a sexually transmitted disease. But it's estimated that about 20 percent of couples seem to pass it back and forth unless both are treated.

Risk factors include excessive moisture, caused by something like sweating or wearing wet clothes, and taking antibiotics, which can kill normal bacteria and allow yeast to overgrow.

Multiple over-the-counter creams and suppositories, as well as oral prescription medicines, are available to treat yeast infections. If getting one of these medicines is impossible, alternatives include:

- **Yogurt:** Put a tablespoon of plain yogurt in the vagina or on the penis daily until the symptoms are gone.

- **Boric acid vaginal capsules:** You can buy these over the counter. Or, if you have some boric acid powder and some 00-size gelatin capsules, open the capsule and fill both sides about half full with the powder. Close the capsule, and insert vaginally. Repeat daily for two weeks.

- **Gentian violet:** Soak a long, large cotton swab in this antiseptic, insert it into the vagina, coat the vaginal walls, then remove and dispose of the swab. Do this daily until the symptoms are gone.

- **Tea-tree-oil douche:** Mix a tablespoon of tea tree oil in a cup of warm water. Douche once or twice a day until the symptoms are gone. Warning: Can cause irritation. Stop if it does.

Warning: Like any treatment, any of these substances may cause side effects in some people. Try a little on the skin of your arm first and make sure it doesn't burn, irritate, or cause a reaction.

Eating yogurt or taking your favorite probiotic may help also. Avoid sugar and alcohol. Diabetes must be under control or the infection is not going away. Also, sex can irritate the area and flair up the infection. Keep the infected area dry by wearing loose cotton clothes and drying well after bathing.

CYSTS

Bartholin's glands are located on each side of the vagina near the opening and secrete fluid to lubricate the vagina. If the opening to one of these glands becomes clogged, fluid backs up and forms a fluid-filled cyst. Sometimes the cyst gets infected and forms an abscess.

A Bartholin's-gland cyst or abscess shows up as a lump or swelling on one side of the vagina near the vaginal opening. It may or may not be painful.

Soak in warm water or apply warm soaks to the area for about twenty minutes every four hours to try to unclog the opening or get the abscess to drain. If the area is tender, antibiotics may be required.

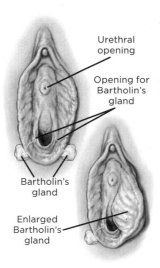

Urethral opening

Opening for Bartholin's gland

Bartholin's gland

Enlarged Bartholin's gland

A clogged opening to a Bartholin's gland can result in a cyst or even an abscess.

Always see a health care professional when possible for a proper diagnosis and to rule out other causes of lumps, such as (rarely) cancer. In some cases the cyst will need to be drained surgically. This might require a lancing with a scalpel and sometimes the insertion of a tube to keep the cyst from filling back up.

BLEEDING

There are multiple reasons for abnormal vaginal bleeding, including hormonal changes, medicines, infections, and cancer. Treating the underlying problem is the long-term solution. NSAIDs may help in the short term.

EMERGENCY CHILDBIRTH

Like the rest of this book, the information in this section is to be used only in the direst of circumstances—at times when no expert is available by phone, by ambulance, by air, or by any other means. Unexpected complications can arise during and after the delivery of a child that can be life-threatening to the mother and the baby. And permanent damage can be done that might have been prevented or lessened in a hospital setting, or at least with a health care worker involved. Having said that, many healthy babies are born to equally healthy mothers every year in emergency situations.

Okay: the contractions have started. They're regular, about twenty minutes apart, and getting closer together. Most of the time, especially with a first baby, you still have many hours to get expert care or for it to get to you. But sometimes, a second or third baby can arrive a lot faster. If the baby's head is showing, or if getting expert help is just going to be out of the question, then what can you do?

Well, ideally, you'll have a partner to help, but back in my pre-med years, when I was working at the local hospital, a wise nurse told me, "Kid, you don't deliver the baby. The mother does that." Good advice to remember, especially if you're ever stuck in a situation where you need to help—or when you're the delivering mother.

Bottom line? In any delivery situation, be patient. Mothers have been having babies for as long as life has been around, often with little or no help at all. And in dire emergency situations, nature will kick in in ways you probably haven't imagined.

So back to the contractions: trying to hurry things along will only cause harm. Slowly, the opening of the cervix will expand from the size of a pinhole to a size that will allow the baby to come out. Slowly the cervix wall will thin and stretch, and the baby will start its outward journey. (Okay, it can be pretty fast sometimes, but the point is, you can't hurry it.)

Preparation

One of the best ways to ensure the health of the mother and baby and to prevent complications during delivery and afterward is for the mother to have regular prenatal checkups. Some potential problems can be prevented, treated early and stopped, or reversed. For others, preparation during or ahead of delivery could lessen the damage. Good nutrition and abstaining from alcohol and tobacco are also essential to limit the risk of damage to the fetus.

SETTING THE STAGE

Unless you already have a pack of sterile equipment, then—just like in the movies—it's time to boil the water and gather some clean towels and sheets. And some scissors or a knife. And two shoelaces or narrow strips of a strong cloth. Boil everything—including the towels, sheets, and shoelaces—for about twenty minutes to sterilize them if you have time. If you can't do that, soak the instruments in alcohol, preferably for twenty minutes or more (three hours is ideal).

Or just do the best you can.

As soon as possible, lay your instruments on a sterile sheet within easy reach of where the delivery is going to take place.

When the Water Breaks

During pregnancy, a baby lives a pretty good life. A thin amniotic sac filled with fluid surrounds the fetus, providing cushioning and keeping bad germs out. The fluid also helps the lungs develop as the fetus breathes it in and out. For further defense against germs, a mixture of mucus and blood plugs the cervical opening.

When things start getting ready to move, the mucus plug uncorks and will come out the vagina. Next the amniotic sac will burst—an event better know as the water breaking. The fluid can come out in a gush or a trickle. Sometimes it's hard to tell the difference between the amniotic fluid and urine. If you're not sure, it's a good idea to check with an expert if possible, because once the water breaks, the baby is at increased risk of infection. That means only rare digital (finger) exams should be performed—and only with sterile gloves—and that the mother should not have sex until after the baby is born (rarely, the water can break several days before labor starts).

Most of the time the sac doesn't rupture until contractions start. Then, or very soon afterward, labor begins. If the amniotic sac is still intact by the time the baby's head is showing (crowning), you can prick the sac with a sterile instrument (your scissors?) and use your hands to remove the film from around the baby's face as best you can.

While you're doing all this, the mother should be sitting, walking around occasionally, sipping some water—doing anything that might help her be more comfortable—and trying to relax. Ideally she's learned breathing techniques: taking a deep breath in and slowly blowing it out through pursed lips during contractions. Encourage her to urinate and move her bowels if she needs to. It's better for her to do this sooner rather than later, for obvious reasons—and it'll make a tad more room for the baby. She, or someone, should be timing the contractions, both how long they last and how much time there is between them.

Prepare a place for the expectant mother, keeping in mind that childbirth is always messy. The towels will be wet from the boiling, but they're going to get wetter. Just make sure the mother stays warm.

SHOWTIME

When the contractions get less than five minutes apart, it's time to start getting ready. The mother needs to have the area around her vagina, rectum, buttocks, and upper thighs washed well with soap and water. A pillow or two, covered with a sterile sheet, should be under her hips so that her pelvic area is raised slightly. That's because when the baby's coming out, he or she will probably be turned sideways while still in the birth canal. The head will need to go down a bit to make room for the upper shoulder to slip out from under the pelvic bone. Have one end of the sterile sheet drape down in front of the mother.

Now it's time for you to wash your hands and your arms, up to your elbows, thoroughly with soap and water. Dry them with a sterile towel. If you have gloves (preferably sterile ones), put them on now.

The mother will usually know when the baby's about to come. Her legs should be spread wide, knees bent, and feet planted firmly. Or she might want to bring her thighs up near her head, holding them with her hands.

Here comes the star.

1. When you see the vagina expanding and a little peek of flesh and hair, the head is "crowning" and you'd better get ready. Again, don't try to rush the baby in any way. It may seem like forever, but no pulling. If the amniotic sac is still intact, this is the time to open it with your sterile instrument. The contractions should bring the baby's head out within a minute or so.

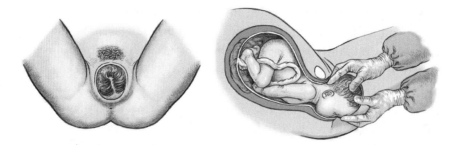

"Crowning" is the first showing of the head through the birth canal. From there, the vaginal opening continues to stretch to make room for delivery.

2. Normally the head will come out facedown. When it's out far enough for you to do so, feel around the neck for the umbilical cord. If it's there, gently and carefully slip it over the head.

3. Hold on to the head to keep it kind of still. But do allow movement. During contractions, the baby's body and head will turn ninety degrees. If anything, slightly help, but mostly wait.

4. When the head and body are at ninety degrees, gently push the baby's head down with each contraction until the upper shoulder slips out from underneath the mother's pelvic bone.

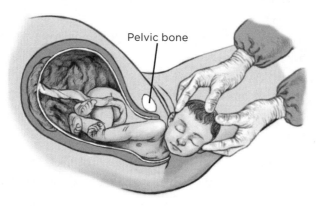

Pelvic bone

After the head is out, gently push the baby down so the upper shoulder will have room to slide past the pelvic bone. Then gently push up so the lower shoulder can slide out. But be sure to get the upper shoulder out first.

5. It should be easy now, so get ready. All you have to do is support the baby as he comes out. Possibly right away or possibly with a contraction or two. Have one hand under the head and neck, being careful not to choke the baby. Keep in mind that he is going to be slippery.

6. When the baby is out, hold him facedown and tilt the head slightly down so any fluids can drain out the nose and mouth. Gently wipe the baby's face with a clean, preferably sterile, towel, and wrap him in a warm, clean blanket.

7. The baby should start crying within a minute. If it takes two or three minutes, perform artificial respiration with your mouth sealed over the baby's mouth and nose. Puff ever so gently.

8. Once the baby cries, hand him to the mother for cuddling and to begin breast-feeding.

WHAT ABOUT THE UMBILICAL CORD?

Of course, at this point the umbilical cord is still attached to the baby. Its other end is attached to the placenta, which is attached to the uterine wall. Just as you did during delivery, take your time here. Never pull on the cord, and never massage the mother's belly to help it come out. When it's ready—and it may take several minutes—the placenta will detach from the uterine wall and come out through the vagina. When this happens, unless expert help is expected really soon, it's time to cut the cord.

1. Get the two shoelaces you've boiled, or tear strips of a sterile sheet. Thin strings don't work well since they may cut into the cord as you tie.

2. Tie the cord about six to eight inches from where it attaches to the baby. The goal is to completely cut off the blood supply from the big artery and vein coming from the placenta to the baby, so tie the cord tightly. Make sure the knot is secure, since if it were to come loose too soon, the baby could lose blood.

3. Next tie the cord tightly and securely again, about an inch farther out from the baby than the first one. This is so that when you cut the cord, not only will the baby not lose blood but also the blood from the placenta won't gush out and make a mess.

4. Using the sterile scissors, or the cleanest you have, cut the cord between the two ties. The part of the cord still attached to the baby should be kept clean and will fall off in a few days.

WHAT ABOUT A BREECH?

If the baby's behind—or even a hand or foot—comes out first, all you can do is be patient. During contractions, you might try to gently readjust the baby's position by having the mother change her own positions or by doing a bimanual adjustment, using one or two fingers inside the mother—while wearing a sterile glove—and your other hand on the pelvis (outside). But without expert help the baby's best bet for survival is mostly making it out on its own.

11

JUST FOR MEN

POP QUIZ

The seventy-year-old man was pacing. He said he'd come to the emergency room because he'd been unable to urinate since early morning. It was 9:00 p.m.

"Have you had any trouble like this before?" I asked.

"No. Well, I mean, I have to stand there for a few seconds before I start, and sometimes I have to strain a little, but nothing like this." He was now shaking his knees back and forth, like a child who really, really has to go to the bathroom.

"Have you drunk any alcohol today?"

He shook his head.

"What about medicines?"

"Don't take any. Well, I did take something for a cold this morning."

"Ahhh."

Which of the following statements is not true?

A. His underlying problem is probably cancer.

B. The immediate treatment is to drain the bladder via a catheter.

C. Either the antihistamines or the decongestants in cold medicine could be causing his urination symptoms.

D. Cold medicines can cause urination problems in women, too.

ANSWERS

A. False. Prostate cancer rarely causes symptoms like this. In fact, many times it causes no symptoms at all. Instead, in men, an enlarged prostate—technically called benign prostatic hypertrophy, or BPH—is the most common cause of acute urinary obstruction. In women, severe urinary retention is less common than in men (incontinence is more common) and is usually a result of nerve or muscle damage during vaginal delivery of a baby.

B. True. The reason the bladder can't empty is the enlarged prostate is pinching shut the urethra—the tube that urine exits the body through. Best case, as the kidneys continue producing urine, the building pressure will eventually force the urine to start leaking out of the urethra, past the big prostate. Even then, sometimes the urine will either get backed up toward the kidneys—eventually filling and injuring them because of the increased pressure—or start leaking into the body from a weak spot in the bladder. In any of these cases, inserting a catheter to empty the bladder is the treatment of choice. Since the urethra is pinched shut, the catheter should be thin in diameter and fairly rigid.

C. True. Cold medicines are a common culprit (see page 210), although many other medicines can cause problems as well.

D. True.

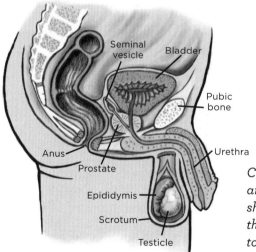

Cross section of the male urinary and reproductive anatomy. Not shown: the kidneys and the ureter, the tube that connects the kidneys to the bladder (see page 181).

ISSUES WITH THE PROSTATE

The prostate is a walnut-size gland that surrounds the urethra. It's adjacent to the bladder and very close to the rectum. It, along with the seminal vesicle, produces the milky white semen that carries sperm.

Portions of the prostate can be felt on a rectal exam. During this exam, the man bends over or lies on his side. The examiner inserts a gloved, lubricated index finger into the rectum. With the examiner's finger fully inserted, palm pointed toward the front of the person, a normal prostate will be felt as a soft, slight bulge about two inches into the rectum.

You can get a feel for the prostate's normal texture by placing your thumb and your index finger together. The little bulge formed in the middle is how it feels. Smooth, firm, but not rock hard.

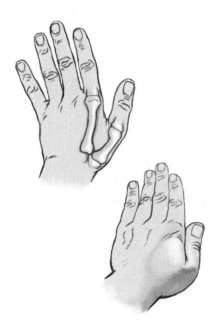

The muscle bulge between your thumb and index finger has a firmness similar to that of a normal prostate on rectal exam.

BENIGN PROSTATIC HYPERTROPHY (BPH)

"Benign" means "not cancerous." "Hypertrophy" means "enlargement." So "benign prostatic hypertrophy" (say that three times fast) means a not cancerous prostate enlargement. Because the prostate surrounds part of the urethra, BPH tends to cause constriction of the urethra.

BPH develops as a normal part of aging, but not everyone has symptoms. And in those who do, the type of treatment often depends on how bad the symptoms get.

Without successful treatment, some people develop acute urinary obstruction, meaning they can't urinate at all. The urine may back up into the kidney and cause kidney damage and eventual failure. When enough pressure builds up, some urine may leak through the bladder opening. Rarely, the bladder wall could start leaking into the abdominal cavity through a weak spot. With or without complete urinary obstruction, if the urine stagnates in the bladder, a urinary tract infection becomes a risk.

Clues that someone may have BPH are:

- Weak urine stream

- Straining to urinate

- Having to stand for a few seconds before urine flow begins

- Dribbling after you think you're finished because the bladder has not been fully emptied

An enlarged prostate may be felt on rectal exam, but because only part of the prostate is accessible to the finger, the exam can be deceiving. Tests performed in a medical facility are necessary for a definitive diagnosis.

Treatment for an enlarged prostate from a health care provider may include prescription medicines or surgery. In one common procedure, an instrument inserted into the urethra cuts away the part of the prostate causing the obstruction. This can also be done with a laser or microwaves, which destroy the obstructive tissue.

There are also a few home treatments and lifestyle tweaks that help many people deal with the symptoms, especially if the prostate is only a little enlarged:

- **Double voiding,** which is urinating, waiting a few seconds, and seeing if you need to urinate again.

- **Trying to urinate regularly:** A full bladder can put pressure on the prostate area and temporarily constrict the bladder opening even more, making it harder than ever to urinate.

- **Avoiding certain medicines:** Antihistamines relax the bladder wall, making it harder for the muscles to contract and force urine flow. Decongestants, even nasal sprays, may constrict the bladder opening. Other medicines may cause problems, so read about side effects and precautions before taking anything.

- **Soaking in warm water** for twenty minutes or applying warm, moist towels to the rectal and scrotal area might temporarily relax the bladder-opening muscles, allowing easier urination. Of course, this assumes that the prostate hasn't fully obstructed the bladder and that there's still a slight opening that, with a little extra urine-flow pressure, will allow urine to leak out (there usually is). If it's been really hard to go, consider urinating while in the water.

Some people also find relief of symptoms with certain dietary supplements that may decrease inflammation and work in other ways to shrink the prostate. Many men rely on:

- Saw palmetto (although its results in clinical studies have been disappointing)

- Rye grass

- Pygeum

- Stinging nettle (which has mixed results in clinical studies)

A diet low in fat and red meat and high in protein and vegetables may help prevent symptomatic BPH.

If you still can't urinate after trying all of these treatments, you may need to use a catheter.

✚ HOW TO INSERT A CATHETER

If someone's bladder must be drained, you've never inserted a catheter before, and you can't get medical help, just finding someone who's done it in the past is much preferable to doing it yourself. But if you're the only one available, make sure you do it in conditions that are as sterile as possible, since introducing bacteria into the bladder is a common complication of catheter use. And to avoid damage to the urethra, be gentle as possible. The damage could also cause swelling of the urethra, making it even harder to insert the catheter.

Because of the length of the urethra in men, and the possibility of a stricture or enlarged prostate, a catheter can be especially difficult to insert in a penis. You'll have to push firmly but not too hard, and you may have to back out a bit and try again, holding the penis at a slightly different angle. The procedure can be very uncomfortable, but if the pain is severe, you're likely doing harm and should stop.

In cases of urine retention, the rigid, narrow, in-and-out type of catheter may be easier to insert. There's also a type called a coudé catheter, which is supposed to be easier to get past obstructions. But the common Foley type may be the only one available. It's little softer but has a balloon on the end to keep it in the bladder.

To insert a catheter, you'll need:

- Sterile gloves and two sterile towels or cloths (boil the towels or cloths for twenty minutes to sterilize)
- A lubricant, preferably one that's water soluble (such as K-Y Jelly or its equivalent)
- Cotton balls soaked with povidone-iodine (Betadine), povidone-iodine pads, or some sort of antiseptic wipes
- A sterile catheter
- A container to catch the urine (or the bag that may be attached to a Foley)

Once you've gathered your materials together:

1. Have the person lie on his back.

2. Position the container so it's ready to catch the urine.

3. Place the sterile catheter, lubricant, and antiseptic wipes on a sterile towel.

4. Place a second sterile towel under the groin area, leaving it sticking out between the thighs.

5. Wipe on and around the urethra with the antiseptics. Start the wipe in the urethra, and make enlarging circles as you wipe outward.

6. Put on the sterile gloves.

7. Pick up the catheter, and coat the tip in the lubricant.

8. Pick up the penis with your nondominant thumb and index finger, and insert the catheter into the urethra.

9. Push firmly and steadily. If there is resistance, back the catheter out an inch or so, readjust the penis up or down a bit, and try again.

10. It may surprise you how far the catheter must go. Remember, the bladder doesn't start until two or three inches past the pubic bone. When the catheter starts draining urine, push it in another inch.

11. Allow all the urine to drain out into the container.

Draining the bladder relieves the immediate problem. But if it fills back up and the person is still unable to urinate, the catheter may need to be kept in place until more extensive medical treatment is available. If that's necessary, a Foley catheter with a balloon is the best type to use.

The Foley has a second small tube running the length of the catheter. This tube has a balloon on it near the tip and a one-way valve on the other end. Once the Foley is inserted, you'll inflate the balloon with water to keep the catheter in. So before inserting it, push sterile water (or water boiled for twenty minutes and then cooled) from the syringe into the balloon and check for leaks. Then remove the testing water and insert the catheter. When urine starts draining, push the catheter in an inch or so more (you never want to blow up the balloon if it's not entirely out of the urethra). Next, push sterile water back into the balloon using the syringe. Now gently tug on the catheter to make sure the balloon keeps it from coming out.

A Foley is sometimes is attached to a bag that will catch the urine. Some types of Foleys actually have a manual valve (separate from the valve that allows the balloon to be blown up) that you can open and close to drain the urine when convenient, so the bag is not needed.

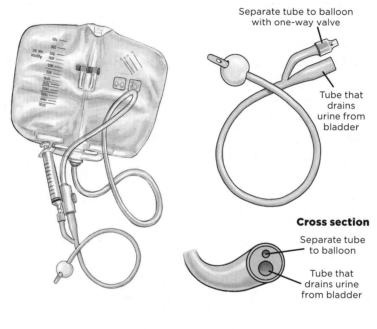

Separate tube to balloon with one-way valve

Tube that drains urine from bladder

Cross section

Separate tube to balloon

Tube that drains urine from bladder

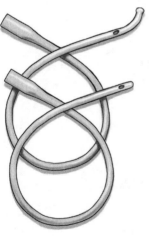

Foley catheter with bag (top left) and without (top right). In-and-out catheter (left front), a rigid, hollow tube with one end flanged (made wider) so it won't go all the way into the bladder. Coudé catheter (left back) is like the in-and-out catheter except it has a narrower, curved, flexible tip that supposedly allows for getting past the prostate easier.

PROSTATITIS

Prostate infection causes even a normal-size prostate to be swollen and tender. When it's touched during a rectal exam, the prostate will feel enlarged and boggy. For the patient, this will feel not just uncomfortable but jump-off-the-table painful. This infection is called prostatitis and is usually caused by bacteria.

In men, back pain, groin pain, and a burning during urination are more likely to be from prostatitis than a bladder infection. So if a man has any of these symptoms, the prostate should always be examined. Sometimes there can also be fever, vomiting, blood in the urine, or a discharge from the penis.

For prostatitis the person will need antibiotics, such as sulfa drugs or ciprofloxacin, for two to six weeks to treat the infection. Limit alcohol and caffeine, but have him drink lots of noncaffeinated, nonalcoholic fluids and urinate regularly. Warm soaks for twenty minutes may relieve some of the symptoms. Ibuprofen or naproxen can help with the pain and decrease inflammation.

If the infection lasts longer than a few weeks, it's called chronic prostatitis. The symptoms tend to come and go. The cause is often unknown, but since bacteria can sometimes be the culprit, two to three months of antibiotics can be worth a try. There is mixed evidence that symptoms may be relieved by periodically massaging the prostate with a finger inserted in the rectum to get rid of a buildup of prostate fluid.

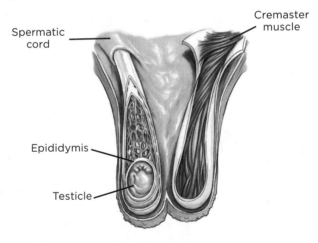

Spermatic cord

Cremaster muscle

Epididymis

Testicle

ISSUES WITH THE TESTICLES

The testicles produce sperm and testosterone. They're covered in a scrotal sac, hang below the penis, and are connected to the prostate and urethra via a tube called the vas deferens.

ORCHITIS

Orchitis is an inflammation of the testicle caused by bacteria or a virus. If it's viral, the mumps virus is the major culprit. Clues that someone may have orchitis include swelling and pain of one or both testicles. Sometimes there's fever, nausea, and vomiting.

If the mumps virus is the cause, symptoms of the regular mumps (painful swelling of the parotid gland in front of one or both ears) typically occur first. Within a few days, one or both testicles get infected.

Orchitis typically lasts three to seven days. If it's caused by the mumps virus (or any virus), antibiotics won't help. Otherwise, antibiotics such as doxycycline or azithromycin are given for two weeks. The person's sexual partner or partners should be treated also.

The following can help relieve the pain:

- NSAIDs

- Bed rest

- Support, such as an athletic supporter or briefs-type underwear

- Ice packs: Hold an ice pack against your testicles for ten minutes, with a towel between your skin and the pack

- Moderate heat: Hold a warm compress or heating pad against your testicles for twenty minutes

- Alternating cold and heat, one right after the other

EPIDIDYMITIS

The epididymis is a thin, extremely tightly wound tube (fifteen to twenty feet long, if stretched out) attached to the back of the testicle. Immature sperm from the testes enter the epididymis and continue to mature for up to a month. When ready, the sperm travel out to the vas deferens, then to the prostate, and out the urethra during ejaculation.

Epididymitis is a bacterial infection of the epididymis. It causes a painful lump in back of the testicle. Sometimes the infection can extend and also cause orchitis, prostatitis, or both. Treatment for epididymitis is the same as the treatment for orchitis.

TESTICULAR TORSION

If the testicle gets twisted, the spermatic cord, which contains the blood vessels that connect to the testicle, also gets twisted, cutting off the blood supply. This condition, called testicular torsion, is painful. Often it's impossible to tell the difference between orchitis and torsion without an ultrasound to see whether blood flow is cut off. If both testicles are involved, or there's fever or mumps, orchitis is likely. Red flags that suggest torsion are:

- Pain after trauma that's not getting better within one hour

- One testicle hanging shorter than the other because that cord is twisted

- No cremasteric reflex (the thin cremaster muscle raises and lowers the testicles, and when the inner thigh is stroked lightly, the cremaster muscle on that side normally raises the testicle; if it doesn't, that's a sign of torsion)

Surgery to untwist the cord performed within six hours of onset almost always saves the testicle. The longer it takes to get to surgery after that timeframe, the less chance there is of saving the testicle. After twenty-four hours, there's little hope. If the testicle dies, it must be surgically removed. In fact the time period is so important that a surgeon may forgo diagnostic tests, thinking it's better to perform surgery needlessly than wait too long.

Occasionally the cord can be manually untwisted and blood flow returned. However, this is risky if it takes time away from getting expert help. And although the cord usually twists in an inward direction, that's not always the case, so you could be trying to untwist it in the wrong direction.

For a cord that's twisted inward, toward the midline, the procedure is to grasp the testicle between a thumb and index finger and twist outwardly. Twist the testicle a full 180 degrees. If this untwists the cord, there will be immediate pain relief. If you're twisting the wrong way, the pain will likely get worse. In that case, you could try twisting the other way. Sometimes you'll need more than one turn to untwist the cord. This can be confusing and tricky, so getting expert help as soon as possible is a much better alternative. Even if the untwisting relieves the pain, the person should be checked by a health care provider as soon as possible to make sure blood flow is good and the cord is in its proper position.

12

KID CONUNDRUMS

POP QUIZ

When my younger daughter was just a toddler she had the croup. Most kids feel bad for a few days, and the virus runs its course. She was different. One night she came into my bedroom. She was coughing, wheezing, and really having trouble breathing. She could barely whisper "Daddy."

I jumped up, pulled on my pants, and sped her to the emergency room a couple of miles away. It seemed like ten. The whole way I was counting her struggled breaths. A couple of times she paused for what seemed like an eternity. I burst into the ER, carrying her in my arms, and yelled at the nurse to call my physician partner. We placed her on oxygen and gave her a breathing treatment, and by the time my partner arrived, she didn't even look sick.

If this happened your child but there was no way you could get expert help, what would be your first step?

A. Take her into the bathroom, turn on a hot shower, close the door, and let her breathe in the steam, far enough away from the shower that there's no chance of a burn. Stay with her at all times.

B. Place her under a blanket or sheet with a vaporizer or steaming water.

C. Have her drink fluids if she's able to.

D. Begin mouth-to-mouth respiration.

ANSWERS

A. Correct. This do-it-yourself steam room would be my first choice. The highly humidified air helps loosen airway secretions, which could be coughed up, allowing better breathing. The earlier this is done the better.

B. Incorrect. The big difference between this steam-tent technique and the bathroom one is you're constantly with the child in the bathroom scenario. Never place anything hot near a child unless you're sure there's no chance for scalding. If you choose the steam-tent method, you need to be under the blanket with the child, holding her in your lap, far enough from the source of heat to prevent a burn, even from the steam.

C. Incorrect. Drinking fluids is a great idea most of the time. It helps keep airway secretions moist and easier to cough up if needed. But I'd be really cautious about offering fluids to a child who is extremely short of breath, because that could invite an episode of choking.

D. Incorrect. The only reason to give mouth-to-mouth respiration in a situation like this is if the child is tiring out completely from the effort of breathing. In that rare case, she may become too fatigued to continue to breathe effectively. The goal of the respiration (no chest compressions!) would be to assist the child until the steam kicked in or perhaps until help could arrive. But remember that kids have smaller lungs than adults do. When doing artificial respiration on a baby, more than a quick puff from you could actually injure the lungs. Seeing the chest rise a bit is evidence that your effort is adequate

CHILDREN ARE NOT JUST LITTLE ADULTS

The simple fact that children are small does have an impact on their health care. For instance, a snake or spider bite is potentially more dangerous in a child than in an adult. But size is just the start of the differences to keep in mind when treating kids.

In children, everything is not only growing but also still developing. This affects how you medicate them, among other things. The still-developing digestive system may not process medicines the same way an adult's does, so be careful never to give a child more than the recommended amount. And just because a medicine is sold over the counter doesn't make it any safer.

Some medicines that are regularly given in adults can cause permanent damage in children. For instance, in children eight and younger, the antibiotic tetracycline can cause permanent teeth staining in the still-developing permanent teeth. Aspirin given with certain viral infections increases the risk of Reye's syndrome, a rare but very serious disease that causes liver and brain swelling. Carefully reading the patient information that comes with every medicine is a must so that you have an idea of what's safe at every age.

Also, never assume that just because something is "natural," it's automatically safe. Raw honey is great for wounds (see page 26), and any real honey can soothe a cough, but honey often contains a few botulism spores—botulism bacteria sealed inside thick, protective walls. The bacteria don't become active until they deem an environment suitable and break out of the walls. In children two years and older, and in adults, the spores just pass through the digestive system, causing no problems. But in children under two, the still-developing digestive tract allows the spores to stick around for a while. Sometimes they'll break through the spore walls, become active, start multiplying, and begin producing their lethal botulism toxin.

Another example of a natural treatment that can be harmful in children is lavender essential oil. Rubbing it regularly on the skin of some prepubertal boys has caused breast enlargement.

There's also mental and social development to consider. Sometimes kids just don't know how tell you exactly what's wrong. If their tummies hurt, they'll point to their midsections almost every time, even if the pain is, say, mostly on the side. And they haven't yet learned the warning signs of things like when they're about to vomit. Sometimes they cry because they're frightened, and other times they seem to ignore the fact they have pain or a serious illness.

So sure, ask them what's wrong, and take their complaints seriously. But in many instances, quietly observing them can better clue you in on how sick they are. If they show no interest in playing or seem irritable; if they're not eating or drinking, or if they just don't look right, something is amiss. If a baby seems to be inconsolable or cries even harder when she's picked up and comforted, that could be a sign that something's seriously wrong.

On the other hand, parents and regular caregivers should also take their intuition seriously. Yes, parents can be overprotective or overworry, especially with a first child. But I've found that sometimes when an exam is normal but the mother just knows something is wrong, her hunch turns out to be right and soon the child starts showing signs of illness. So when a caregiver tells me something's up but I can't find anything, I always tell her to continue to keep a close eye out for new signs of problems.

CHILDREN'S BONE AND JOINT INJURIES

Children's bones are more flexible than adult bones—kind of like young pine trees versus aging oaks. This can be a good thing. I've seen many a child's hand that has been slammed in a car door. This injury normally crushes the bones in an adult. But often in a child there's only a bad bruise. And even if a child's bone is broken and crooked, many times it will straighten as it heals.

On the other hand, children's bones have growth plates. If one of these plates is injured badly enough, especially if the plate is slightly displaced, the growth of the bone can be severely stunted, or the bone can become deformed.

So have injuries checked out by a health care provider, especially if discomfort is not going away in a day or two. Injured growth plates need to be realigned as perfectly as possible. You're really not going to be able to do that without expert care. But in the absence of professional help, if a bone in an extremity is injured, splint it as is (see page 42). Even if the bone is crooked, it often may heal normally. At a minimum, try to avoid further injury and movement until the bone has time to heal. See Chapter 3 for more specifics on treating bone and joint injuries, especially if there's swelling or displacement that could injure nerves or arteries.

FEVER

Usually, a fever means infection. And kids get lots of those. Most infections are viruses, so antibiotics don't help. Children's immune systems fight them off in a few days, and everything gets back to normal—most of the time. But even run-of-the-mill infections can have complications.

If a child feels bad, is not eating, or is not behaving normally, he may not be able to communicate what the problem is. One of the best tools in your figure-it-out arsenal is a thermometer. If he's running a fever, an infection is the likely issue.

On the other hand, many kids run a fever and never miss a beat. Even in that case, you should slow your child's activities down. As it does in adults, the immune system fights best if it's not competing for energy or running low on fluids.

Also, a good rule to know is that with many infections, the fever gets higher in the evening. Many people feel pretty good in the morning only to feel like mush by nightfall. So until a child has a fever-free evening, he's not over the infection.

Nursemaid's Elbow

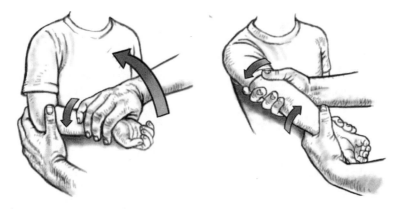

Putting a nursemaid's elbow back in place

Nursemaids get a bad rap on this one, because nursemaid's elbow can happen when anyone—not just a nanny—picks a young child straight up by the hand or hands. The pulling can cause a bone in the elbow (the radius) to slip out of place ever so slightly. Swinging a child around by the arms can do it as well, dads.

Nursemaid's elbow is a young child's injury—age five or under. At that age, the ligaments holding the bone in place are still a little loose. The injury can also occur with a fall, but a break is more likely in that situation.

The child usually cries in pain for a few minutes, then stops but won't use the injured arm. Any attempt to move it brings back the pain and crying. Until you can get treatment, try applying an ice pack (with a cloth held between skin and pack) for about ten minutes at a time. Sometimes the bone will just go back into place by itself, but waiting for that when it may not happen could result in swelling, stiffness, and difficulty in treatment. On the other hand, if the injury is causing a lot of real pain (not just fear), then there may be a crack or tear, and the best thing to do might be just to leave it alone.

If and when you can get to a health care provider, she'll probably do an exam and X-ray. If there's no break, she'll put the bone back in place like so—never forcing any movement:

1. Get the child's mind on something other than the injury. The procedure shouldn't hurt much, but the child will be scared.

2. The child will be holding the arm, slightly bent at the elbow. Slowly twist the forearm until the palm faces upward.

3. Bend the elbow to the max.

4. Straighten the arm.

And that's it. Feeling or hearing a pop is a suggestion of success, but the main evidence that the procedure worked is that the child will be able to move his arm without pain.

To be extra safe, consider having the child wear a sling for about a day if he's willing.

FEVER IS NOT THE ENEMY

Fever in itself is not a bad thing. When your body is invaded by germs, one way it fights them is by increasing your core temperature. Most germs thrive within a certain temperature range, so your body is trying to change the environment so the germs won't thrive as well. Only if a fever gets close to 106 degrees Fahrenheit is it potentially dangerous. The point is, don't obsess over getting the fever down. Take it as a warning sign of an underlying infection, and that infection should be your focus.

That said, one of the side effects of fever is discomfort, and that can be a reason to try to bring it down. The main health risk is that the person will be so miserable that he won't drink enough fluids and will become dehydrated. And dehydration can be a killer.

Bottom line: fever tells you something's wrong. Look for the cause and treat it appropriately. In the meantime, make it a priority to have the person drink fluids.

BRINGING THE FEVER DOWN

If you do want to bring the fever down, certain medications, such as acetaminophen, will usually help, as will a lukewarm bath or sponging with lukewarm water. But never, ever give more than the recommended dose of medicine, and never give it more often than directed. Also, never bathe anyone in cold water or with alcohol. The shivering it causes can make the body temperature rise even higher.

In fact, overall, keep a feverish child warm but not too warm. Don't bundle him up more than normal. If the child is sweating, either the fever is coming down (you can check to see) or he's too bundled up. Chills can be a sign that the fever is going up.

WARNING SIGNS

If there's fever, look at the child overall to try to figure out how serious the illness is. Does he look sick? Is he drinking fluids? Playing? Drinking and playing are clues that the infection may not be that bad. Still, remember that kids can go from looking fine to being very sick in nothing flat. So keep a good eye out for changes.

Here are some of the reasons to consult a health care provider as soon as possible:

- A child is three months old or less and has a rectal temperature of 100.4 degrees Fahrenheit or higher

- Any child's temperature rises to around 106

- The fever is above 103 and won't come down to at least 101 with medicine or sponging

- A child has a petechial rash (see page 227)

- The fever is accompanied by a severe headache or stiff neck, which could indicate meningitis, a serious infection of membranes that surround the brain and spinal cord

- A child is getting dehydrated (see page 225)

- A baby won't stop crying, which may be the only clue you have that something is seriously wrong

- You're just really worried, even in the absence of the above signs and symptoms.

Meningitis

Meningitis is a worry for many parents because this serious infection hits children, up to the teen years, the most—and because it can cause life-threatening complications.

So far in this book, I've mentioned meningitis as a potential cause of a seizure (page 81) and as a possible complication of an ear infection (page 118). Meningitis can also be spread like a cold: via saliva or nasal secretions, such as through coughing or sneezing. That's why if even a single case happens in a dorm, military barracks, or a school—or in an emergency shelter—it becomes a big worry.

Meningitis will usually cause fever, but of course any infection could cause fever. More specific clues are severe headache and a stiff neck—any neck movement causes pain. That's because meningitis causes an inflammation of the meninges, which is the covering of the spinal cord. In babies, the only signs may be fever, looking really sick, and being inconsolable. In fact, any touch usually causes more crying. A definitive diagnosis can only be made with a spinal tap done by a doctor.

CAUSES

Bacteria, viruses, and, less frequently, fungi may cause meningitis. Some viral meningitis infections are very serious and need to be treated with hospitalization and antiviral medicine. But many viral cases are no worse than a really bad cold or flu and are gone in a couple of weeks without any treatment other than rest and staying hydrated.

However, with bacterial meningitis (and some viral cases) the results can be devastating. Brain damage, hearing loss, and death are a few of the complications that occur. For the bacterial type, intravenous antibiotics and other expert measures are needed to treat the infection and prevent the complications. For the less common fungal infections, treatment involves antifungal meds.

The only way to know for sure what type of meningitis you have is through a spinal tap performed by a doctor. So get to a doctor if you possibly can.

PREVENTION

A person with meningitis can be contagious for up to a few days before symptoms begin. Handwashing and avoiding crowds are two of the most effective preventive measures, along with getting vaccinated.

The three most common causes of bacterial meningitis are pneumococcus, haemophilus, and meningococcus bacteria. Most people get the pneumococcus and haemophilus vaccines in childhood. The meningococcus set of shots may be taken as an option sometime between ages 10 to 25, but the immunity does tend to start weakening after about four years. A booster is available.

Taking a certain type of antibiotic can decrease your risk if you've been in close contact with someone with bacterial. Check with your doctor if that's an option.

SWOLLEN LYMPH NODES

It's been my experience that the immune systems of healthy children work great—maybe better than adults'. One example is the lymph nodes. They're those glands in the neck and other places that swell and get tender when they're trapping infections coming from other parts of the body—including the throat, ears, sinuses, and skin. In children, the lymph nodes have a tendency to become very large and tender when fighting infection—a sign that they're doing their job really well. And since lymph nodes are located all over the body, even in the abdomen, a viral infection or strep throat can often cause abdominal pain. As the infection resolves, so does the abdominal pain.

Note: I've had many patients tell me their tonsils are swollen—and then they point to the lymph nodes in their neck. (See the illustration.) When these particular lymph nodes swell up, the infection is likely (though not always) located above the neck. But it's not necessarily tonsillitis. The problem could be in the ears or sinuses, for example.

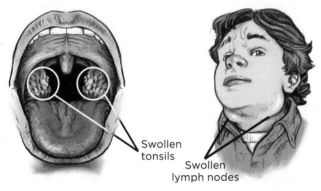

Swollen tonsils

Swollen lymph nodes

Some people confuse swollen lymph nodes in the neck for tonsils. Tonsils are composed of lymph node tissue, but they're located in the back of the throat. Infected tonsils usually cause swollen lymph nodes, but swollen lymph nodes don't have to be from infected tonsils.

DEHYDRATION

Children can get dehydrated quickly. In many countries dehydration is a leading cause of death. Vomiting or diarrhea can lead to dehydration. So can not drinking enough fluids—which is easy to do when you're feeling bad.

The signs of dehydration can be subtle. They may include lethargy, infrequent urination, the absence of tears when crying, a dry mouth and tongue, a sunken fontanelle (that soft spot on a baby's skull), and eyes sunk back in the sockets a little more than normal. For treatment options, see page 186.

RASH

A rash is like a fever in that it's a sign of, or clue to, an underlying problem. Some infections, especially viruses—such as chickenpox and fifth disease—are known for their type of rash. Often, when a kid gets a rash and feels sick, you'll find that one of these infections is going around. Figuring out what other kids in the area have could help you identify the infection. In developed countries, a rash-and-fever combination in children is typically caused by a virus that will run its course. Of course, a virus always carries a chance of serious complications, but treatment usually consists of rest and fluids. Also watch for signs of possible complications, such as increasing lethargy, signs of dehydration, or just looking worse in general.

As a rule, if a rash itches, a warm shower or bath makes the itching worse and makes the rash look more pronounced. Be aware that this effect is temporary and not dangerous.

THREE WORRISOME RASHES

Three rashes to be particularly concerned about are the scarlet fever strep rash, petechiae, and hives.

Scarlet fever, or scarletina, is caused by the streptococcus bacteria. This infection brings a sore throat (known as strep throat), usually fever, and a typical strep rash. The rash spreads over most of the body and feels like fine sandpaper. Because scarlet fever is bacterial, antibiotics, such as amoxicillin, cephalexin, or azithromycin, are recommended. Before antibiotics, this infection was often a killer. And antibiotics dramatically decrease the risk of rheumatic fever, which can otherwise occur after a strep infection.

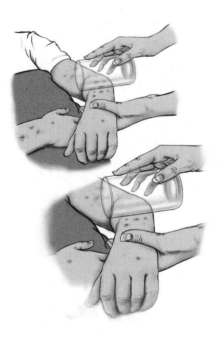

The glass test: when you press the skin with a clear glass, petechiae don't fade.

Petechiae are small red or purple flat dots, splotches, or blood blisters. They actually consist of blood that's leaked out of small blood vessels close to the skin surface. The rash doesn't itch and doesn't blanch, or fade, when pressed on. It can be a warning sign of a very serious infection and should be checked out by a health care provider if at all possible.

Life-threatening viruses, bacterial infections, and sepsis are some of the worrisome causes of petechiae. On the other hand, straining from hard coughing or vomiting can sometimes break a few of the tiny blood vessels around the face. This is nothing to worry about. But since many of the diseases that cause petechiae require strong intravenous medicines, unless you're sure the petechiae are a result of too much straining, get expert evaluation as soon as possible.

Hives, which are patchy, irregular, raised, and splotchy, suggest an allergic reaction. They often itch and may occur on any area of the body. The patches can be larger than the usual spotty rash. They range in size from less than an inch in diameter to several inches in diameter. An antihistamine or prescription oral steroid may help, depending on the age of the child. Avoiding the medicine, food, or whatever caused the reaction is key. If there's any associated shortness of breath or swelling of the throat, neck, or face, immediate expert care is essential, along with an injection from an EpiPen Jr, a prescription medicine you should ask your doctor for in advance and store in your first aid supplies.

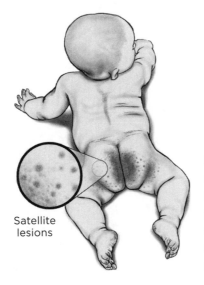

Satellite lesions

Satellite lesions are small spots scattered beyond the main area of diaper rash and suggest the cause is a yeast infection.

DIAPER RASH

Just about anything that touches the skin can cause an irritating rash on the exposed area. Many diaper rashes are irritant rashes. Some potential irritants are urine, feces, chemicals, and diaper chafing. Bacterial and yeast infections can also be culprits. To treat or prevent a diaper rash, change the diaper often and keep the baby's bottom clean and dry. Your favorite soothing cream or a little over-the-counter hydrocortisone can also ease the symptoms. Aloe vera gel is a good alternative. If the baby develops little satellite lesions, a yeast infection should be suspected, and an antifungal cream may help.

13

THE ELEMENTS

POP QUIZ

On one of the few occasions when I've played golf, it began to thunder in the distance. I was a young teen and had never heard the expression "When thunder roars, go indoors," but I knew from my lifeguard experience that thunder meant lightning, so I headed off the fairway.

I took a shortcut through some woods. Just as I was crossing a barbed-wire fence, lightning struck. I heard a boom, and I felt a strong tingle in the hand that was touching the fence. I don't know if it was the electricity or my adrenaline, but the next thing I knew I was lying down on the other side of the fence, heart beating fast but no worse for wear. Looking back, I realize the wire could have been just charged with nondangerous static electricity from the lightning, but I learned a thing or two.

True or false:

A. If you hear thunder, lightning can strike, even if the sky is clear.

B. When there's lightning, you're not safe anywhere outdoors—not in the clear, in the trees, or in a golf cart.

C. A shed or a cave provides protection from lightning similar to that of a house.

D. When you're in a car, the rubber tires protect you from lightning.

ANSWERS

A. True. Lightning can strike you from a cloud more than ten miles away. Since ten miles is just about the maximum distance you can hear thunder, that should be a definite warning sign that you're at risk.

B. True. If you're outside, there's no safe place from lightning. But we also know that lightning likes to strike the tallest object in its path, so if there's no way to get into a safe shelter, such as a house or a car, some experts recommend squatting in the middle of a low-lying clump of medium-size trees. If you're in a group, spread out.

C. False. Inside a fully enclosed car (not a convertible) or a house is by far the safest place to be. Lean-tos and small shelters are not. Neither is a cave or under a rock ledge. Lightning can travel through wood and rock. If you're in a house, stay away from windows. Also avoid plumbing, electrical wires, and phone wires—and anything attached to them. In a car, roll up the windows and don't touch any metal. Don't use your cell phone, since the current could travel through it to you.

D. False. Rubber, either on the soles of your shoes or on tires, is no match for lightning. It's the metal frame around the car that protects you, because most of the electrical current stays within it.

LIGHTNING AND ELECTROCUTION

Feeling your hair standing on end is a telltale sign that lightning is about to strike. You may also hear hissing, high-pitched, or crackling sounds or see a blue halo around metal objects (which you should be away from anyway). This means that electrical activity is building up.

Quickly leave the area if you can. Some experts suggest that if shelter is not available, you should just keep on walking, and if lightning strikes odds are one of your feet will be off the ground when it does. Another suggestion is to crouch down on the balls of your feet with your heels close together. Keep your head down and your hands off the ground. The theory is that if you're struck, the electrical current won't be as likely to pass through your whole body. How much this technique really helps is a matter of debate.

If you do get struck by lightning, a large amount of electricity will course through your body. This can burn flesh, damage nerves, and even stop your heart. At least the burns aren't usually severe or deep. Small comfort if your heart's stopped, but many people do avoid that particular side effect and survive lightning strikes. If you're wearing metal, though, you may find a severe burn at the metal site because the heat from the current localized there and charred you. Then again, many times there's no burn at all—from metal or anything else.

Another thing you may discover is that you're missing clothes. The lightning sets off a shock wave from the blast of electricity. The sudden, powerful blast of air can knock your clothes off, throw you around, break bones, and burst eardrums.

After a lightning strike, you'll probably feel dazed and confused. In addition to burns and musculoskeletal injury, lightning can cause:

- Temporary blindness from the light

- Temporary deafness from the blast waves

- Varying degrees of amnesia

- Severe headache

Lightning isn't the only potential cause of electrocution during a storm—or on a sunny day. Other causes could be touching a live wire or stepping in water that's connected to one.

If someone is struck by lightning or electrocuted in any way and has no signs of life, call for help if you can and start chest compressions (see page 141). The one caveat is to make sure you don't get electrocuted, too. The current from a lightning strike leaves the victim's body almost immediately, so there's no danger of your getting shocked by touching her. But if the victim has been electrocuted by a wire—in standing water or not—you're going to have to disconnect the wire from her body or from the water or move the person without getting electrocuted yourself. Possibly you could use a wooden stick or some nonconductive tool, but that's risky. You might be able just to turn off the electricity. Or you may not be able to do anything unless expert help arrives with special equipment.

If there's an automatic external defibrillator around, use it. If the victim is unconscious but breathing and has a pulse, protect her from the elements as best you can, but otherwise leave her alone. There could be broken bones that vigorous moving would damage.

If the victim is conscious, the evaluation is much easier. Try to calm her down if she's agitated or confused. Splint any suspected fractures and get her to shelter.

Anyone struck by lightning should seek expert care as soon as possible. Even if everything seems okay, long-term problems such as depression and pain can set in later.

THE ELEMENTS

EXTREME HEAT

Most of your essential organs reside in your body's core. The organs there operate most efficiently at 98.6 degrees Fahrenheit, give or take a degree or two. So your body constantly works to maintain this temperature. If its regulating mechanisms get overwhelmed, you need to correct the problem soon, or it could become life threatening.

To cool off your body, your blood vessels dilate (get larger), bringing warm blood close to your skin, where its heat can be released into the air. You also produce sweat, and when it evaporates, it cools down your skin, allowing heat to escape a little faster.

Heat-related problems—anything from feeling a little too hot to developing heat exhaustion to having heatstroke—fall on a spectrum called hyperthermia. If you catch the symptoms early and cool off, you can often reverse the progression. But if you wait too long, the process may become an irreversible death spiral.

PREVENTION

Wear loose, breathable clothes and a wide-brim hat. Do any heavy outdoor work before 10:00 a.m. and after 4:00 p.m. Take frequent breaks in the shade. Fan yourself a little. Since an early sign of heat exhaustion can be confusion, work with a partner, or at least have someone check on you periodically.

Drink a couple glasses of liquids per hour, because dehydration makes hyperthermia worse. Avoid excessive amounts of caffeine, sugary drinks, and alcohol. If you're performing manual labor outdoors, you need as much as a quart or two of liquids per hour. The drink doesn't have to be ice-cold. In fact, too-cold liquids can cause stomach spasms. If you're drinking water, add a teaspoon of salt to the first couple of quarts each day, unless your doctor has suggested limiting your amount of fluids or salt. In that case, get his or her advice about what to do. For examples of additional suitable beverages, see page 186.

If you're inside with no air-conditioning, open windows and use a fan. Good ventilation is essential. However, when the temperature gets in the high nineties, though fans may make you feel more comfortable, they cannot cool off your body temperature. There are three ways fans can cool you: by evaporating sweat, moving hot air away, or directing cool air in. When the temperature is extremely hot, the fan is just moving hot air around, and evaporating sweat isn't enough to cool you to a safe temperature. Also, high humidity can make it difficult for sweat to evaporate. High temperatures and high humidity can be especially dangerous for people whose bodies don't adapt well to the heat anyway, including elderly people, kids younger than four, and people with certain chronic illnesses. Instead of a fan, what does work is a cool midday shower, bath, or sponging. Or here's an old trick: putting a bowl of ice in front of the fan cools the air it's blowing on you.

HEAT EXHAUSTION

Heat exhaustion occurs when your body is no longer able to cool your core. It's your last warning: unless you immediately stop generating extra internal heat (exercising) and cool off externally, you may progress to heatstroke. In fact your mechanisms for trying to stay cool have become so exhausted that your core is already starting to overheat.

Warning Signs

Heat exhaustion can cause:

- A sudden, massive increase in sweating
- Muscle cramps
- Extreme weakness
- Dizziness
- Headache
- Confusion
- Pale skin color
- Low blood pressure
- A pulse rate well above one hundred
- A weak pulse
- Fainting
- Nausea or vomiting
- Goose bumps and skin that's cool to the touch

Treatment

If you suspect heat exhaustion, stop work immediately. Not when you get to a finishing place; not in a few minutes. Immediately. Your body generates heat with activity.

Find the coolest spot available, and lie down. Drink some liquids. People with heat exhaustion are almost always dehydrated. The fluids will help cool you and help your circulation work more efficiently to cool you off.

Stay cool and don't work the rest of the day. Your body needs time to recuperate.

HEATSTROKE

This is a life-threatening emergency. Your cooling system has gone beyond exhaustion and no longer works at all. Yet your metabolism—the chemical reactions your body produces that enable you to stay alive—generates heat constantly. So your organs basically begin cooking. Not good. It's a difficult, sometimes impossible problem to overcome, especially outside of a medical facility.

Clues

One of the first organs that shows damage from heatstroke is the brain. Therefore, many of the signs and symptoms of heatstroke are related to brain function:

- Agitation
- Euphoria
- Confusion
- Seizure
- Hallucinations
- Coma
- Disorientation

Non-brain-related signs of heatstroke include flushed skin, severe headache, no sweating at all, a fast heart rate, and rapid breathing.

Treatment

Call 911 immediately if possible. Never wait to see whether someone with heatstroke is going to get better on his own, because even if you fully hydrate and cool someone with heatstroke, he'll have damage to multiple organs.

Until the ambulance arrives, cool the victim off as best you can. If he can walk and it's not far, get him into air-conditioning. Otherwise have him lie down in the shade. Take off all but his underclothes. Spray or bathe him with cool or cold water and fan him. If the victim is unconscious, place him on his side so his tongue won't impede his airway.

If there's no way to get expert medical help, your only hope is to cool the victim off as quickly as possible and get some fluids into him. If you have access to cool intravenous fluids, and the training to use them, now's the time to give them. In addition:

- If you have ice, place a pack on the victim's groin and armpits and under his neck. As always with ice packs, place a cloth between the skin and the pack.

- Experts disagree about whether someone with heatstroke should soak in a tub of ice water. The problem is, if his heart stops, it's going to be difficult to do

CPR. I'm of the opinion that whatever gets him the coolest the quickest is what you should do.

- Soak a sheet in the coolest water possible and wrap it around his bare skin.

- Fan him for the cooling effect of evaporation.

- If he's alert enough, have him slowly drink as much cool water as possible.

PRICKLY HEAT, A.K.A. HEAT RASH

Sweating a lot can clog sweat glands, which could then become inflamed and show up as a rash in the affected area. This is more common in children, whose sweat glands are still developing, but it can happen to anyone. And it's not just a nuisance. Clogged glands don't produce effective sweat for cooling, which increases the risk of hyperthermia. They can also get infected.

Clues

Heat rash shows up as small, itchy, red bumps in areas that are prone to getting hotter than other areas—often the back, neck, or face.

Treatment

Rub ice on the rash for a few minutes, and keep the area open to the air. Wear loose, cotton clothes so your skin can cool and the sweat evaporate. To try to unclog the pores, take frequent showers or baths, but to avoid irritating the skin, use a mild soap, and don't scrub hard. Lanolin can help.

EXTREME COLD

Cold-related problems, like heat-related problems, fall within a spectrum in which the symptoms range from mild to life-threatening. And when you're cold, just like when you're hot, it's important to keep from getting dehydrated. Hydration enables your circulation to work efficiently in its quest to regulate your core temperature. But since you're usually not sweating when you're cold, your hydration needs may be easier to forget. Also, because confusion can be an early sign of hypothermia, it's just as important in cold weather as in hot to have a partner so you can monitor each other.

PREVENTION

To prevent hypothermia, dress in layers, stay out of the wind, and stay dry. One of the reasons to dress in layers is so you can take some of them off if you start sweating.

Keep yourself fueled properly, too. Stay hydrated, drinking warm, noncaffeinated drinks if available. And eat plenty of snacks. If your body is trying to stay warm, it's easy to deplete your energy-essential carbohydrates. Your body uses food the way a fire uses wood—as fuel to produce heat.

Now, here's what *not* to do:

- **Don't drink alcohol.** Alcohol dilates your surface blood vessels and brings blood to your skin at the expense of your vital organs. You *feel* warm, but your heart, liver, and kidneys are suffering. Alcohol also impairs your judgment. The combination of alcohol (or other mind-altering drugs) and cold weather is a major killer every year.

- **Don't rub your skin to warm up.** Vigorous rubbing dilates those surface vessels in the same way alcohol does.

- **If you're indoors,** don't start a fire or turn on a fuel-burning space heater or stove without adequate ventilation. Wood, paper, coals, gas, oil—you name it—burning any organic material produces carbon monoxide, which can poison and kill you. (Electric space heaters or stoves don't pose a carbon monoxide threat, though you'll of course want to take precautions to make sure they don't overheat or trigger a fire.)

MILD HYPOTHERMIA

Mild hypothermia occurs when your body is really working hard to keep your core warm. If you don't help it out, at some point it's going to tire and become less efficient.

Mild hypothermia can cause:

- Shivering
- Trouble thinking
- Confusion

- Deteriorating judgment
- Forgetfulness
- Fast heart rate

Treatment

Put on more layers of clothing, stay dry, and stay off the cold ground. Drink fluids, warm ones if available. And eat something. Your body needs fuel to generate heat.

MODERATE HYPOTHERMIA

Your body is giving out by the time it has moderate hypothermia. Soon all the mechanisms it uses to keep you warm will malfunction. You need external heat, and you need it quickly.

Shivering stops with moderate hypothermia. You become more confused, and you may even start taking off your clothes because you think you're warm (it's a weird reaction to hypothermia called paradoxical undressing). Your heart rate may slow and become irregular. You're at risk for life-threatening heart rhythms.

Treatment

Follow the treatment for mild hypothermia. Build a fire or get inside. If you have heating pads, place them under your arms.

Be gentle when treating someone else. At a cold body temperature, the heart becomes very sensitive and can go into dangerous rhythms with too much jostling.

If you're getting really, really cold and there's no other way to get warm, two or three people can get under blankets, take off their clothes, and get skin to skin. It's worth a try. And no, don't use this as a ploy to get lucky!

SEVERE HYPOTHERMIA

When you have severe hypothermia, your body is no longer conserving heat and is generating less heat than normal. The essential organs are cold, and the heart is very sensitive. Minor irritation can trigger a deadly rhythm.

A person with severe hypothermia is unconscious or very hard to awaken. The pulse is weak, and breathing is becoming shallow.

Treatment

One of the keys to treating an unconscious person with hypothermia is to get to a place that has advanced warming techniques, such as warmed IV fluids, warmed breathing devices, and just plain heat. At the same time, keep yourself safe. If you're out in the middle of a frozen nowhere, you can expend only a finite amount of time and energy before you put yourself in danger of exhaustion and severe hypothermia.

FROSTBITE

When the liquid in your skin and in the underlying fat and muscle cells freezes, ice crystals form, cells dehydrate and die, and blood vessels are damaged. Depending on how deep the freezing goes, this can result in blisters, sloughed-off dead skin, deep tissue damage, or gangrene.

Frostnip is a big red flag that frostbite's coming. It happens just before the liquids freeze and causes tingling and numbness. At this stage, the skin is irritated, but rewarming before it freezes can prevent skin damage.

With longer exposure to the cold, the outer layer of the skin becomes frozen first. From there the deeper layers begin to freeze. Eventually the skin becomes white and frozen. As deeper tissue freezes, it becomes numb and hard.

Before treatment, take off any restrictive jewelry or clothing, because warming will probably cause swelling. Then immerse the area in warm water—around 100–108 degrees Fahrenheit. The tissue should thaw within fifteen to thirty minutes. If you don't have a thermometer, you can test whether the water is too hot by sticking your uninjured hand in it. You shouldn't have to remove it. Keep the water moving a little. It helps keep the warmest water next to the injury. Keep the temperature constant, or more skin damage may occur. Be very gentle with the damaged tissue. Let the injured area air-dry. Don't towel-dry or rub.

Expect swelling, large blisters, and severe pain. Those are signs the tissue is rewarming. Don't prick blisters, even the large ones, unless they're already leaking. A sealed blister is a sterile environment and limits infection risk.

After warming the frostbitten area, dress the wounds: get some absorbent padding, such as gauze or cotton, and coat one side of it with an antibiotic cream. Silvadene (1 percent silver sulfadiazine) is a good one. Neosporin (or another "triple antibiotic"), gentamicin, and bacitracin are alternatives. When applying the dressing, place it between fingers and toes if they're affected. Make sure the dressing isn't so tight that it restricts movement or blood flow. Take into consideration that the wound may swell. To reduce swelling, keep the injured area at heart level or above.

You may want to try aspirin or ibuprofen (Advil, Motrin) for pain, if you have them, since they provide additional frostbite-related benefits that aid in healing: they decrease inflammation and increase circulation a bit. Also consider taking a vasodilator (a medicine that dilates the blood vessels, allowing for increased blood flow, which could help in healing). Some blood-pressure medicines help if you're already on them. The B vitamin niacin is worth a try if you don't have ulcers. (Niacin may make your skin flush and tingle.) Don't smoke. Smoking constricts blood vessels. Start antibiotics, if available.

Don't walk, stand, or put pressure on the injured area any more that you absolutely have to until the wounds have healed. If you have to walk in the cold for help and the risk for refreezing is high, don't start warming the frostbitten area until you reach your destination. There tends to be less permanent damage from frostbite if you don't have to rethaw.

CARBON MONOXIDE POISONING

Any source of heat that requires burning produces carbon monoxide fumes in the process. Coal, any kind of gas, alcohol, paper, candles, wood, charcoal, you name it: if you're burning it, you should have adequate ventilation. And don't think that just because you can't see carbon monoxide or smell it it's not there. The gas is odorless and colorless, and its effects come on gradually. Headache and drowsiness are common symptoms, but many people die in their sleep.

CLUES

Suspect carbon monoxide poisoning if you find someone unconscious or extremely drowsy in a poorly ventilated enclosed area (room, tent, vehicle . . .). Carbon monoxide poisoning is especially likely if you see evidence of previous or current fossil-fuel burning. The evidence could be in the room or just outside it—for example, a generator within fifteen feet of the structure could be the culprit.

The cherry-red lips that are often described as a classic sign are rarely seen. In fact, there's no definitive physical sign that screams out, hey, this person is unconscious due to carbon monoxide poisoning! The circumstance you find the victim in is your main clue.

TREATMENT

Carbon monoxide attaches to your red blood cells in place of life-giving oxygen. To get his oxygen back, the victim must stop breathing carbon monoxide and begin breathing oxygen—the purer the better.

Transfer the victim outdoors. Give him pure oxygen if you have it, but since that's very flammable, remember to first snuff out any open flames. If you can't transfer the victim outside, open the windows and doors, and get rid of the source of the fumes. And, of course, call for expert help if it's available.

WHEN WATER IS SCARCE

No matter the situation, you're not going to survive long without fluids. If, thanks to a natural disaster or a terrorist attack, your water supply is contaminated or cut off for days, you're up a really dry and dangerous creek. So when you're amassing your survival supplies, water is one of the first things you should stash away plenty of.

If you have some warning before an emergency, filling your bathtubs from the tap is a great idea. But really, whatever's in the tubs should be thought of as extra, because you may not get that warning in time to fill them—and you may need much more than your tubs can hold.

How much should you store? On average, every person is going to need about two quarts a day for drinking—more if it's really hot or if you do much physical exertion. Factor in your needs for hygiene, cleaning wounds, and other necessities, and a gallon per day per person is the minimum. Two is better. Even if your storage area is small, try to store at least six gallons per person total. If you have the room, I'd suggest twenty gallons or more.

If you buy commercially bottled water to store, heed the expiration dates. Tap water is fine to store as well. The chlorine in it helps keep the germs out. Consider rotating stored tap water every six months or so—drinking the old and replacing with new. (If you reuse the water bottles, clean them thoroughly first.) If you keep the tap water around longer than that, though, it really should be fine if it's sealed. Just to make sure it's drinkable, you could use some of the disinfection tips (page 241).

Certainly other beverages, such as milk, juice, sports drinks, and sodas, can substitute for drinking water. Ideally, you should use them only as a supplement to water. They may not be as well digested or may contain too much sugar or salt. Of course if you have a scarcity of food, the sugar could be a short-term plus. And depending on the type of drink, you might get electrolytes and vitamins.

MAKING WATER DRINKABLE

If, during an emergency, you only have access to untreated water, in most cases your main interest should be disinfecting it—killing the germs. But if toxic chemicals are a problem, things become more complicated. For example, if you're drawing water from a stream that's contaminated with factory runoff, disinfection won't get rid of the chemicals. For that you need to distill the water (see page 244) or use charcoal filtration (see page 244). Even then, though, there's no guarantee that all chemicals will be removed.

HOW TO DISINFECT WATER

No matter which disinfection method you use, if the water is cloudy, first strain it through a clean piece of cotton fabric or a coffee filter. This removes debris and some bacteria. Then let the water sit for a couple of hours to allow residual sediment to settle. Pour all but the sediment into a clean container.

Boiling

Bringing water to a rolling boil should kill all the germs in it, but by letting it boil for a minute or two you can be sure the water's disinfected. Use a lid if you have it to keep the water as hot as possible and to keep some of that precious resource from evaporating away.

Chlorine

Chlorine kills viruses and bacteria, but it may not kill all the parasites, such as giardia and cryptosporidium—they're carried in some animal feces, which often contaminates streams and lakes.

Add two to four drops of unscented 5.25-percent chlorine bleach (such as regular-strength Clorox) to each quart or liter of water. That's eight to sixteen drops per gallon. Mix it well. Wait thirty minutes or so before drinking it.

If you're using calcium hypochlorite granules (often used to disinfect swimming pools), it's a two-step process. First mix your starter: one teaspoon of the granules dissolved in two gallons of water. Store this starter solution and label it "bleach—NOT FOR DRINKING." It should stay good for about two weeks. Next add one part of this bleach solution to one hundred parts water. That equals:

• Two teaspoons of bleach solution to one quart or liter of water

• Eight teaspoons of bleach solution to one gallon of water

• One pint of bleach solution to twelve and a half gallons of water

Mix well and let sit for thirty minutes before drinking.

Iodine

Don't disinfect with iodine if anyone who will be using the water is allergic to it. Also, like chlorine, iodine may not kill all parasites.

Add one of any of the following items to each quart of water (for a gallon of water, multiply the quantities by four):

- 1 iodine tablet
- 5–10 drops 2-percent iodine solution
- 8–16 drops 10-percent povidone-iodine (Betadine) solution
- 1–2 small povidone-iodine (Betadine) pads

Mix well and let sit at least thirty minutes before drinking.

UV Rays from the Sun

To disinfect water using the sun's ultraviolet rays, first ensure that the UV rays can get to all the germs: the water should be at least clear enough to read a newspaper through. If it's not that clear even after filtering (see page 241), mixing a quarter teaspoon of salt into every quart or liter of water can help. But be aware that this is about six hundred milligrams of sodium and could overload someone on a salt-restricted diet. A typical low-sodium diet usually includes no more than two thousand milligrams per day. Some people should consume even less.

Then disinfect: put the water into a clear plastic bag, mason jar, or plastic bottle that holds no more than two liters. Seal the container, and place it on its side in the direct sun for six hours—forty-eight hours if the sky is really cloudy. Adding about a quarter teaspoon of 3-percent hydrogen peroxide or about an ounce of lemon or lime juice per liter of water can shorten the time the UV rays take to kill the bacteria.

Microfiltration

Backpackers and hikers often travel with a portable microfilter that allows them to remove microscopic organisms from their drinking water. I recommend keeping a microfilter on hand for emergencies. When choosing one of these devices, make sure the manufacturer guarantees that it has no pores (holes) larger than one micron. Microfiltration is better than chemicals at removing parasites, but since viruses can be smaller than one micron, they might get through. So combining this method with the chlorine or iodine method described above is ideal. However, many filtration systems do come with a layer of activated charcoal, which will catch a lot of the escaped viruses.

Getting the water through the microfilter will require gravity or some other force, such as sucking the water through a special filtered straw. All microfilters should come with directions.

HOW TO MAKE A SOLAR STILL

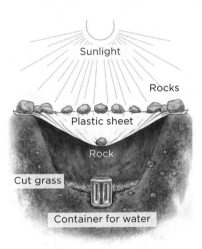

A solar still will draw water from the ground and certain other sources, such as plants. You'll need a container to catch the water and a large clean plastic tarp.

Dig a hole in the ground around four feet in diameter and three feet deep, or larger if you can. Just make sure the hole diameter is small enough that the plastic tarp can seal it off. Dig a little well in the center of the hole and place the water-catching container in it.

To add moisture, place any available green vegetation in the hole—this could include grass, leaves, and vegetables. If you have a flexible, clean tube long enough to allow you to suck the collected drinking water from your container, you won't have to unseal the hole and lose valuable moisture every time you need a drink.

Cover the hole with the plastic tarp and weigh down the edges with rocks, dirt, or both. Use as much as necessary to seal it and keep the plastic from blowing open in the wind.

Place a rock or dirt or both in the middle of the plastic so that it droops down into the hole about forty-five degrees. The bottom of the plastic should be centered over the water container.

Over a period of several hours, moisture from the ground and the vegetation will rise, be caught by the plastic, condense, and drip back down into the container. The cooler the plastic, the faster the condensation, although the plastic should remain above freezing.

This solar still method should produce drinkable water. It might not be completely free of disease-causing germs and chemicals, but chances are good that it's better for you than undistilled contaminated water.

You won't be able to get a great deal of water from a solar still. How much you get depends on how much moisture is in the ground and in the vegetation you use. You could even place dirty water, seawater, or urine in a separate pan in the hole and allow its condensation to drip down into your clean bowl as well.

HOW TO REMOVE CHEMICALS FROM WATER

Activated Charcoal

Activated charcoal, also known as activated carbon, has a slightly positive charge that makes certain chemical molecules stick to it. This process is called adsorption. In addition, the activation process gives the charcoal millions of pores of different sizes, which tremendously increase the charcoal's surface area so more liquid can come into direct contact with it. The pores are actually too large to filter out 100 percent of bacteria and viruses, so you'll need to combine activated charcoal with a disinfectant method if you want to make sure you get rid of germs as well as chemicals. Moreover, since activated charcoal works well on some chemicals but not others, you'll need to find out which toxins may be in your water and whether activated charcoal will remove them.

Activated charcoal comes with some portable water bottles and faucet filters. You can also buy it separately. It's used for fish tanks, too.

Since chemicals stay stuck to activated charcoal, you'll have to replace the charcoal regularly. How often you need to do this depends on how much water you filter and how contaminated it is.

Distillation

Not only does distillation get rid of many toxins, it also kills germs. You can purchase a commercial distillation system or make your own. Overall, distillation ensures the purest drinking water, but even then it can't remove all types of chemicals. And because it also removes minerals, good and bad, some experts believe that drinking only distilled water long-term might carry its own health risks.

The basic premise of distillation is that different liquids have different boiling points, and many are higher than water's. So with this method, you boil water and catch the steam. The chemicals that have a higher boiling point than water will be left behind, as will minerals and other solids. The steam will condense back to a purer water.

Here's one simple distillation setup:

1. Choose a big heatproof container and fill it about one-third full with the contaminated water.

2. Place a brick or similarly sized, flat heatproof object inside the filled container.

3. Place a smaller clean heatproof container on top of the brick. The small container should be tall enough to stand clear of the splashing of any contaminated water. The brick is meant to help with the height.

4. Place a lid upside down on the larger container so that the convex side faces down.

5. Boil the water.

Steam will collect on the inverted lid. As the steam cools and condenses back to water, it will drip into the smaller container. The cooler the lid, the faster the steam will condense, so you can put ice on the lid if you have some.

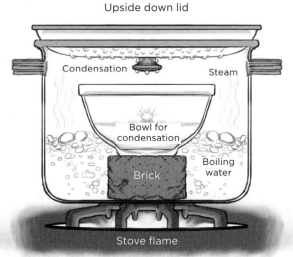

Upside down lid

Condensation

Steam

Bowl for condensation

Boiling water

Brick

Stove flame

Because distillation requires boiling for a while, it kills bacteria, viruses, and parasites. If done properly, distillation can remove about 99 percent of many pollutants, but it can't be counted on to remove chemicals that have a boiling point around or below that of water. Examples include toluene, benzene, and some pesticides. These products will turn to steam along with the water and end up in the second, "purified" container.

According to the United States Environmental Protection Agency, products that contain toluene include gasoline, paints, synthetic fragrances, adhesives, inks, and cleaning agents. Benzene is found in gasoline, coal and oil emissions, industrial solvents, and tobacco smoke.

DRINKING SEAWATER, URINE, AND BLOOD

People often ask me whether they can drink last-ditch fluids such as seawater, urine, and blood. These may hydrate you for a very short time but are so concentrated with other ingredients, including toxins, that in the long run your body will lose more water trying to dilute them and excrete the toxins via your kidneys than you will gain by drinking it. You'll become more dehydrated than you would by drinking nothing at all. However, distilling seawater and even urine will remove many of the concentrates and make these fluids drinkable (see page 244).

14

THE SURVIVAL DOCTOR'S SUPPLY CLOSET

POP QUIZ

As I said in Chapter 1, preparation is essential to surviving disasters of any kind. By reading this book, you've just finished the most important preparation of all—you've gathered the knowledge you'll need to handle any situation. But there are only so many medical treatments you can give with your bare hands. To aid most health problems, you need supplies.

Someone once asked me what my number-one piece of survival equipment would be. My answer? Duct tape.

It's true! Duct tape can be a lifesaver. After reading this book, you know that duct tape can help remove a wart, close a wound, and make a tourniquet. But there are many other amazing medical uses for duct tape. Which of the following is *not* something you can do with duct tape?

A. Make eyeglasses—lenses and all.

B. Protect your skin from waterborne diseases during a flood.

C. Filter germs from water.

D. Stop a lung from collapsing.

ANSWERS

A. Incorrect. See page 111 for instructions on how to make pinhole glasses with duct tape.

B. Incorrect. Wrap the tape around some old shoes or boots and up your pant legs as far as you need. Make sure it's not too tight and there's no space where the water could leak. Warning: The tape may damage your clothing as it is taken off.

C. Correct. Duct tape is a wonderful tool, but since it is waterproof, it can't be used as a filter.

D. Incorrect. You can tape and seal an open chest wound or fold the sticky sides together and make it into a one-way valve as described on page 151.

PROTECTING THE HEALER

"First do no harm" applies not only to helping to a victim. It applies to the one doing the helping as well. In fact, if you get sick or hurt, you're not going to be helping anyone. That's why those flight attendants always advise putting on your oxygen mask first. And it's the reason for using personal protective equipment.

You may opt to store more than the following suggestions, depending on your level of expertise, worry factor, and budget. Just remember that no matter how many gloves and masks you have, you have to wear and dispose of them correctly if you want to keep germs at bay.

NONSTERILE GLOVES

Tips: Since some people are allergic to latex, consider nitrile or vinyl disposable gloves. Vinyl gloves are a little less sturdy, but you can always wear two pairs. Get a size that fits all. A little large is better than too small. For the car and go bags, you could place a few in a plastic bag.

Substitutions: A plastic bag could be used as a barrier as a last resort. Ordinary nondisposable household gloves, intended for chores such as washing dishes, are good and tough but might be difficult to disinfect after every use.

STERILE GLOVES

Sterile surgical gloves are more expensive than nonsterile gloves. But it's important to use them when tending to burns and to wounds that involve broken bones.

MASKS

Tips: I recommend storing two types of masks: surgical masks and N95 respirator masks. Surgical (or dust) masks are more comfortable, so you can wear them longer. But their pores are too large to ensure protection against viruses. It's better if they're worn by the infected person, because they at least keep germs from getting sprayed everywhere through coughs and sneezes. N95 masks protect against 95 percent of infectious particles but must be fitted with a complete seal around the mouth to protect properly. They can be very uncomfortable to wear for more than a few minutes. So you can wear one while you're treating someone and then remove it (with your gloves on) when you're at a safe distance. N99 respirator masks protect even more (99 percent of infectious particles) but are denser and can be even more uncomfortable, so it's more tempting to break the seal to get a little relief.

Substitutions: A scarf or other material tied around your face (or the sick person's) is better than nothing as long as it doesn't impede breathing and oxygen intake.

FACE SHIELD OR GOGGLES

Tips: Both face shields and goggles protect your eyes from bodily fluids and from solid foreign bodies when you're cutting wood or grinding metal. However, if the goggles fog over, you may be tempted to use your contaminated hands to adjust them. Face shields aren't sealed all the way around but are more comfortable.

Substitutions: Eyeglasses of any sort protect at least a little.

PROTECTIVE GOWN AND SHOE COVERS

Tips: Disposable protective gowns and shoe covers usually aren't necessary unless you're caring for someone who has a dangerous contagious disease that involves explosive diarrhea or vomiting, or you're treating someone whose blood might splatter onto you.

Substitutions: Any waterproof plastic could serve as a gown and shoe covering. Even a raincoat might do in a pinch.

DISPOSABLE BARRIERS WITH ONE-WAY VALVES

Tips: While administering artificial respiration, a little one-way-valve mouth barrier comes in handy. It allows your breaths through but blocks the victim's secretions. You can even buy these as keychain attachments.

Substitutions: A plastic bag or a glove with a hole cut in it is better than nothing, but makeshift solutions don't provide that one-way valve protection.

CLEANERS

Store plenty of soap to use for personal hygiene. Keeping your skin clean is even more important than usual when you're in a survival situation. Also, I like to store things that can be used for more than one purpose, such as the following disinfectants.

- **Rubbing alcohol (also called isopropyl alcohol):** This is good for sterilizing instruments and, if you have no clean water, for cleaning wounds and washing hands. It stings on wounds, though.

✚ HOW TO MAKE YOUR OWN SURFACE DISINFECTANT

Mix one cup of 5.25-percent chlorine bleach (such as regular-strength Clorox) in nine cups of water. Or mix one teaspoon of calcium hypochlorite crystals (like the ones used to disinfect swimming pools) in two gallons of water and let sit for thirty minutes. Then measure one cup of that mixture and add it to nine cups of water.

Pour the solution on the area to be disinfected (such as the countertop or floor) and let it soak for thirty minutes. Then wipe dry with a clean cloth. For all cleaning and mixing, leave the windows open for fresh air, and use waterproof gloves, a mask, goggles, or a face shield—and, if possible, a disposable covering for your clothes—to avoid coming into contact with either splashes or fumes from the solution or germs from the surface you're disinfecting. Both cleaning solutions will deteriorate with time, so pour them down the drain after no more than two weeks.

- **Povidone-iodine (Betadine) pads:** Use these to clean around wounds or to disinfect water (see page 241). A bottle of povidone-iodine instead of the pads is fine but potentially messier. Povidone-iodine has been found to be pretty effective in preventing rabies if it's used to irrigate away the bacteria in an animal-bite wound soon after it occurs.

- **Bleach:** Household bleach—5.25 percent—can be used to disinfect surfaces (see previous page) and water (see page 241).

BANDAGES AND DRESSINGS

Adhesive bandages (Band-Aids): Keep a few of the regular and large sizes in your medicine cabinet and go bags.

One-ply gauze rolls (such as the Kerlix brand): You can cut some to size for a dressing, fold it over to make it thicker, wrap it around an extremity to make a pressure dressing, or use it to secure a splint around a leg or an arm.

Nonsterile gauze pads (or sanitary napkins will do): I like the three-by-three-inch or four-by-four-inch sizes. I'd buy a big box of them, place a few in resealable plastic bags, and store the bags in each go bag and first aid kit.

Sterile gauze pads: These usually come in individually wrapped packages. They're more expensive than the nonsterile kind, so you can save them for burns, wounds involving broken bones, and other injuries that have a high risk of bad infection.

Nonstick sterile gauze pads: Keep a few of these individually sealed squares in each kit. They come in handy for placing on a burn or a wound that might continue to ooze blood or other fluids. The nonstick quality helps keep the fluids from drying and sticking to the bandage, which can then be painful to pull off. The downsides are that this type of gauze is more expensive and because it's not as porous, it doesn't sponge up wound fluids as well as regular gauze.

Tampons: You can use these to apply pressure to nosebleeds, puncture wounds, or for any place they fit to help provide pressure to stop the bleeding.

Elastic bandages (such as ACE): The three-inch and four-inch widths are the most versatile. They come in rolls and with metal or Velcro clips.

Self-adherent elastic wrap: This is also known as Coban, vet wrap, or Ve-trap. It's a kind of elastic bandage that clings to itself, but it's not readily reusable.

Cotton balls soaked in petroleum jelly (Vaseline): These can be stored in resealable plastic bags in your small first-aid kits. Petroleum jelly can help seal a dressing for a chest puncture wound or make it easier to insert nasal packing when treating a nosebleed. It can also remove hot tar stuck to the skin. And the soaked cotton balls make great fire starters.

Adhesive tape. Any tape can be used to secure a bandage or close a wound (see page 24). Duct tape is waterproof and has many nonmedical uses, but the glue on it can irritate the skin. Be sure to keep some latex-free tape around in case you're treating someone who is allergic to latex.

QuikClot or Celox gauze: These products use chemicals to clot bleeding that can't be stopped with pressure or a tourniquet, including bleeding from wounds located too high up in the thigh or arm to leave room for a tourniquet. The products only work if they come into direct contact with the bleeding blood vessel. Often, more than one package is needed to pack the wound. If you buy QuikClot, purchase the gauze version—the older, granular type is harder to completely clean out, which you must do before the skin of a wound is closed.

Israeli bandage (a.k.a. emergency bandage): This can be used as a pressure wrap or a tourniquet. It's easy to learn how to use, but make sure you do so before you need it. (It comes with instructions, or you can find them online.)

Bandage scissors or all-purpose scissors: Keep a good, sturdy pair of these blunt-tipped scissors in your car, go bag, and home emergency kit.

Unstick a Bandage

If a bandage gets stuck to a wound, pour some sterile water or povidone-iodine (such as Betadine) between the wound and the bandage. Then let it soak for a few minutes to see if the adhesions will loosen.

USEFUL EQUIPMENT

Thermometer: A digital or nonmercury oral model is fine.

Stethoscope: Listen to some normal lungs and hearts before an emergency arises.

Blood-pressure cuff: This is bulky, and really, feeling a pulse with your fingers—noting its rate and whether it's weak or strong—can tell you enough in the field. But a blood-pressure cuff can help you monitor whether a person's blood pressure is trending lower or higher. This could help you assess whether someone in shock is getting better, and it could help you know how much blood pressure medicine you should be taking. A manual cuff in particular can also be used as a tourniquet or pressure dressing. For home, consider an automatic cuff because it's easier to use. The kind that fits over your arm tends to be more accurate than the kind that fits over your wrist. Verify the device's accuracy by letting a trained person check your pressure with a manual cuff, then check it again with the automatic one.

Pulse oximeter: Clip this device to a finger to painlessly determine the oxygen saturation in the blood. It also measures pulse rate. It's helpful, too, in discerning shortness of breath from a panic attack, a condition in which the saturation will be close to 100 percent. You can also use it to help determine whether heart and lung problems need immediate treatment and supplemental oxygen (see page 152).

Tourniquet: Any strong, flexible material about an inch wide and long enough to tie or twist around the extremity can be used as a tourniquet, but many emergency experts warn to not take chances. A commercial tourniquet can sometimes stop bleeding when makeshift items can't.

SAM Splint: Structural, aluminum, and malleable, a SAM Splint consists of padded strips of aluminum than can be fitted to work as a neck brace or splint any joint other than the hip and shoulder.

Cervical collar: This is nice to have and doesn't take up much space, though the SAM Splint is a great alternative.

Slings: Stock up on child and adult sizes, though you can usually come up with an alternative for these in a pinch. One trick I like is safety-pinning the bottom of your shirt high enough to provide a pocket to cradle your arm at about a ninety-degree angle.

HOW TO STERILIZE EQUIPMENT

None of the following procedures is a guarantee that all germs will be killed. But they may be your best alternatives outside of a medical setting if you don't have sterile prepackaged supplies on hand.

First, clean off debris with soap and water or rubbing alcohol. You may need a cloth or brush. Then use one of the following cleaning agents.

Pressurized steam: If you have a pressure cooker, know how to use it properly, and have the time, this can be the best method for disinfecting metal instruments and even cloth. Place the objects to be disinfected on a rack above the water level and use a PSI of fifteen or more for thirty minutes or longer. Of course, be careful. That hot steam can cause a bad burn.

Boiling water: Submerge the equipment in a container of boiling water for twenty minutes. Partially cover with a lid, if available, to keep the heat high.

Fire: If you're disinfecting a metal object, hold the part that's going to touch the injury over an open flame. If the handle is also metal, find something to hold the instrument with so you don't burn your fingers. Heat until the metal turns red; that's long enough. Then let the instrument cool, and you're ready. If I have rubbing alcohol on hand, I like to dip the instrument in it afterward just for good measure.

Chemicals: If the above options aren't possible, soak the instruments in povidone-iodine, chlorine, or alcohol for twenty minutes or longer. If that's not an option, wipe the instruments off with a clean cloth soaked in one of those solutions.

ADVANCED EQUIPMENT

Emergency airways: These devices keep the back of the tongue from obstructing the airway in an unconscious person. You need a variety of sizes, and you need to know how use them (see page 159).

10-ml syringes: These can be used to irrigate wounds. If you have a needle and the expertise, you could also inject intravenous, intramuscular, and subcutaneous medicines. The syringes are useful for measuring liquid medicines, too, which you can then squirt directly into the mouth. I'd keep five syringes in each emergency kit.

Urinary catheter: A Foley catheter can be useful when you need to drain a bladder (see page 211) and even to treat certain types of nosebleeds (see page 123). The device's diameter is measured in a unit called a French (Fr). One French equals one-third of a millimeter. On average, a 14 Fr or 16 Fr usually works well, but for emergencies in which blockage can be a problem, an even smaller 12 Fr wouldn't be a bad idea. Urine might leak around it once it's in place, but it should be easier to get in the bladder. Another catheter option is the in-and-out type. It has no balloon to keep it in, but it tends to be narrower and stiffer than the Foley. In addition to a Foley, it's nice to have a bag and tube that connect and drain the urine without a mess.

NONMEDICAL EQUIPMENT

Headlamp: This comes in handy when you need both hands to do a medical procedure.

Flashlight: Make sure to stock up on extra batteries.

Paracord survival bracelet: This is a strong cord with multiple uses that's braided into a bracelet.

Emergency blanket: A wool blanket gives the most heat insulation. A sleeping bag is bulkier, but of course it might be better for camping. Heat-reflective aluminum-coated blankets are the lightest but not good insulators. They work best if you place the shiny side next to your body and add a coat, blanket, or other form of insulation on top. You can also use one as a tarp to reflect heat to you from an external source. Don't forget gloves and a hat.

Safety pins: Have various sizes available for occasions when you need to pin elastic bandages or make slings. You can also use a pin to stick a hole in the bottom of a plastic bag or jug to make water pressure for pressure cleaning a wound. If you use it for picking out splinters, sterilize it first if possible.

Matches and/or lighters: Keep these in a waterproof case. Use them to start a fire or sterilize needles, safety pins, scissor tips, and so on.

Eyeglasses: Keep an extra pair on hand.

Superglue: This substance, sold under several brand names (such as Super Glue, Gorilla Glue, and Loctite), is especially good for small finger nicks, which could lead to big infections in a dirty environment. It can also be used to close small wounds. Superglue can be irritating, so test it on uninjured skin first.

Supplies for water purification (see options on page 240).

Clean containers, such as pots and resealable jars: You'll need something for boiling water, storing your homemade disinfectant (see page 250), distilling water (see page 244), and so on.

Pressure cooker: Store one of these if you want to use it for equipment sterilization (see below).

MEDICINES

Keep medicines in waterproof, crush-proof containers if you're traveling. All medicines are best stored in dry, cool conditions. A thermos or ice chest might help protect them from swings in temperature. And periodically replace your supply. Here's a tip for that: when you get new medicine, put it in your first aid kit and use the older medicine from the kit instead. Before using any medicine, whether prescription or over-the-counter, read the package insert and note the dosages, side effects, interactions, and warnings. The guidelines below are only partial.

OVER-THE-COUNTER MEDICINES

I recommend keeping a few individual packets of the following over-the-counter medications in each first aid kit. Stock up on liquid or chewable versions for the kids, too. The items in this list are just suggestions. Customize according to your own needs and preferences.

- **Ibuprofen** (Advil, Motrin), **naproxen** (Aleve), or **acetaminophen** (Tylenol) for pain and fever relief—remember these are often included in pain and cold medicines, so don't overdose

- **Diphenhydramine** (Benadryl) for allergies or to use as an occasional sleep aid

- **Ranitidine** (Zantac), **famotidine** (Pepcid), or your favorite antacid for heartburn and acid reflux

- **Loperamide** (Imodium) for diarrhea

- **Nasal decongestant spray,** such as oxymetazoline (Afrin), to restrict blood vessels during a nosebleed

- **Hydrocortisone cream 1-percent** (Cortaid) for eczema, poison ivy, poison oak, and any other noninfectious skin irritations
- **Miconazole cream** (Monistat) or another yeast-infection medicine
- **Clotrimazole cream** (Lotrimin) for jock itch or yeast infections
- **Permethrin lotion** (Nix) for scabies
- **Pyrethrin shampoo** (Rid) for head or pubic lice
- **Antibiotic ointment:** I like bacitracin; **triple-antibiotic ointment** (Neosporin) is fine, but some people are allergic to it; raw honey is a great alternative for people two and older
- **Multivitamins:** If you can't get fruits and vegetables for an extended time, these could come in handy to prevent vitamin deficiencies; the chewable kids' type could be a great option for everyone, and keep a sealed bottle of the prenatal type if there's a chance of pregnancy
- **Neem oil** for head lice, pubic lice, or scabies; this may also repel mosquitoes
- **An aloe vera** plant (see page 31) or a bottle of aloe vera gel for burns and for soothing the skin
- **Lidocaine gel** for numbing a wound before you clean or suture it
- **Petroleum jelly** (Vaseline) for sealing in the skin's moisture if you don't have lotion; it's also about the only thing that gets tar off skin, and it can help seal chest puncture wounds (see page 151)
- **Raw honey** for eating and coughs, and to use as an antibacterial ointment in people two and older (see page 26)
- **Medihoney,** a type of honey known for its antibiotic properties that's been irradiated to ensure that it contains no botulism spores (so it should be safe for small children)
- **Clove oil** for toothaches
- **Tea tree oil** for poison ivy, lice, and scabies and for fungal infections of the skin, such as jock itch and athlete's foot
- **Activated charcoal,** which can be used for water purification (see page 244) but may also be effective in treating certain cases of poisoning (see page 189)

PRESCRIPTION MEDICINES

Always refill prescription medicine a few days early so you'll never run out completely. Also you could ask your prescriber for a little extra to keep on hand just in case. She might have some free samples or be willing to prescribe you a month's extra. You'll have to pay out of pocket for the latter, but if you take a generic medicine, it may be cheap.

EpiPen

Also ask your doctor if she'll prescribe you an EpiPen. This is epinephrine in an automatic, self-injecting container. Keep it readily available to grab at a moment's notice in case of a life-threatening allergic reaction. It could also be used for a severe asthma attack if you don't have an inhaler. (Also keep an EpiPen Jr on hand if you care for children.) As soon as you purchase your EpiPen, open the box and read the instructions so you'll know how to use it before you need it. Quick use could mean the difference between life and death.

Antibiotics

It's somewhat controversial to include antibiotics in this list. One the one hand, antibiotics are often the only things that will save a life. On the other hand, they're complicated to use—there are dozens of types, and you need to know the right one for your problem—and they can have side effects—sometimes serious ones. Beyond that, antibiotics don't work against viruses, and often even doctors can't tell whether an illness is viral or bacterial without a laboratory test. Overuse has contributed to bacterial resistance: some bacteria have mutated to the point that antibiotics no longer kill them. This is having a potentially devastating impact on our world.

Nevertheless, if you wish to store antibiotics, your doctor might give you a prescription for at least one round to keep in your emergency medical supplies. Antibiotics must be stored in a cool, dry place. They'll be labeled with an expiration date. Usually, most of them will last a lot longer, but temperature extremes and humidity can alter their potency

Only use your stored antibiotics when you absolutely need them and cannot get to a doctor for diagnosis and prescription. Take the full round—all the doses that are recommended—so that you're sure to knock out the bug rather than leave a few stragglers to mutate into bacterial resistant versions. And I reiterate: read labels and precautions. The guidelines below are by far not complete.

Commonly used antibiotics include:

- **Azithromycin** (Zithromax, Z-Pak): Can treat strep throat, ear infections, sinus infections, bronchitis, pneumonia, whooping cough, skin infections, and chlamydia

- **Amoxicillin:** Great if you're not allergic to penicillin, but many bacteria, such as staph, have become resistant to it; cephalexin is a good alternative

- **Ciprofloxacin** (Cipro): Good for bacterial gastrointestinal infections, but only take it if the infection is severe or won't go away; it's also good for prostatitis, urinary tract infections, and gonorrhea; it may cause abnormalities in anyone whose bones are still growing (typically 18 and younger); don't use it if you're pregnant

- **Metronidazole** (Flagyl): Treats the internal parasite giardia and the sexually transmitted parasite trichomonas; makes you deathly sick if mixed with alcohol

- **Sulfamethoxazole/trimethoprim (Septra, Bactrim):** Good for urinary tract infections, and this combination antibiotic is one of the only oral meds that treats community-acquired methicillin-resistant staphylococcus aureus, or MRSA; don't use it if you're if pregnant or allergic to sulfa meds

- **Ivermectin:** Kills many intestinal-worm infections, including pinworms; also kills scabies and body, pubic, and head lice; don't take it if you're pregnant, breast-feeding, or younger than six years old

- **Mupirocin** (Bactroban): a prescription antibacterial ointment or cream to use on wounds; kills many types of bacteria, including staph, strep, and MRSA (over-the-counter antibacterial ointments help prevent infections but don't actively kill bacteria)

PROFESSIONAL SUPPLIES

If you have appropriate hands-on training, add the following supplies.

IV MATERIALS

- **A bag of IV fluids,** such as lactated Ringer's solution
- **An IV kit**

• **Needles,** including catheters, butterfly-type infusion sets, intraosseous infusion needles (which stick into a bone so the fluid can travel the same route as the bone marrow; many paramedics say these are the easiest to use in a non-hospital emergency setting)

SUTURE KIT

• **A suture holder**

• **Small scissors,** to take the sutures out

• **Suture with a needle connected:** 3-0 or 4-0 nylon (Ethilon) should be strong enough to hold most wounds together

• **Local anesthesia (for numbing):** Lidocaine solution, 1 or 2 percent, is what medical personnel use, but it's prescription, and you'll need syringes and needles for it; lidocaine gel or ice packs and other options have variable results

Or, instead of the suture holder, scissors, and suture with needle, you could opt for skin staples and a skin staple remover, which tend to be a bit easier to learn how to use.

ADDITIONAL ADVANCED SUPPLIES

• 14-gauge, two-inch-long hollow needle for chest air-pressure release (see page 153)

• Orophangeal airways (OPAs), which prevent an unconscious victim's tongue from occluding the airway (see page 159); it's best to get a package of various sizes because the fit is important: the tip should go past the tongue but not too deep into the airway

• Nasopharyngeal airways (NPAs) of various sizes: These are generally easier to use than the OPAs because they're inserted through the nostril (see page 160), so you don't have to deal with opening the mouth and getting by the tongue; they're also less likely to make a semiconscious person gag

INDEX

G

gallbladder attacks, 173–174
gallstones, 175–176
gas pain, 177
gastritis (stomach irritation), 174
gastrointestinal infections, 185–189, 258
gauze rolls and pads, 251
gauze substitute, 24
gentian violet, 199
germ protection, 9
giardia, 259
ginger, 119
glass test, 226
gloves, 248
goggles, 249
gonorrhea, 258
gowns, protective, 249
growth plate injuries, 220
gunshot wounds, 151–152, 166–168

H

haemophilus vaccine, 224
hallucinations, 75, 234
hands
    animal bites to, 99
    fractures, 54–55
hand washing, 11
hawthorn extract, 133
headache
    after head trauma, 79
    fainting and, 85
headlamps, 254
head lice, 256, 257, 259
headstands, 126, 137
head tilt, 157
head trauma (concussion), 78–80
head wounds, 25
heart, heart problems
    anatomy, 135
    blood clots, 139–141
    blood pressure, 131–134
    cardiac syncope (fainting), 84
    chest pain, 126–131

CPR for, 141–143
    fast heart rate, 134–137
    heart attack, 126–127
    vs. panic attack, 137–139
    quiz, 125–126
    supplements for, 133
heartburn, 256
heart rate check, 135
heat-related problems
    altered mental status, 74
    heat exhaustion, 233
    heatstroke, 234–235
    prevention of, 232–233
    prickly heat (heat rash), 235
Helicobacter pylori, 175
hepatitis, 172
hepatitis B vaccine, 4
hernias, 183–185
hip and thigh fractures, 57–58
hives, 227
hobo spiders, 96
hollow needles, 260
honey
    child safety warning, 26, 219
    as eyedrops, 109
    for wound care, 26, 257
humerus (upper arm) fractures, 47
hydrocortisone cream (Cortaid), 256
hygiene, 10, 11
hypertension, 131–134
hyperthermia, 74, 232–235
hyperventilation, 92, 149–150, 152
hypothermia, 74, 236–237
hypovolemic shock, 87

I

ibuprofen (Advil, Motrin), 196, 256
ice, applying to injury, 2, 41
ice-water facial, 137
immunity building, 3
immunizations, 4
Imodium (loperamide), 256
incarceration (hernia), 185
incisional hernia, 184

staph infections *(staphylococcus aureus),* 16, 258, 259

steam, for sterilization, 255

steam treatments, 156

sterile gauze pads, 251

sterile-gauze substitute, 24

sterile gloves, 248

sterilization instructions, 202, 255

steroid creams, 10

stethoscopes, 252

stinging nettle, 211

stomach flu, 185–189

stomach irritation (gastritis), 174

stomach pain. *See* abdominal pain

strangulation (hernia), 185

strep *(streptococcus)* bacteria, 16, 259

strep rash, 226

strep throat, 224, 226, 258

stroke, 76, 80

stys, 110

Sudafed (pseudoephedrine), 156

sugar, for wound care, 26

sulfamethoxazole/trimethoprim (Septra, Bactrim), 259

sunburn prevention, 10

sunlight
    for disinfecting water, 242
    solar still, 243

superglue, for wound care, 21–22, 254

supplements
    for asthma, 155
    for enlarged prostate, 211
    for heart problems, 133
    for menstrual cramps, 196

supraventricular tachycardia (SVT), 126, 134–137

surface disinfectant, 250

surgical masks, 249

suture kit, 259–260

suture substitutes, 24–25

SVT (supraventricular tachycardia), 126, 134–137

swelling, 42

syringes, 253

T

tachycardia, 126, 134–137

tampons, 251

tar removal, 30

tea tree oil, 257

tea-tree-oil douche, 199

tension pneumothorax, 152–153

testicles, testicle problems, 214–216

tetanus shots, 4

tetracycline, 219

thermometers, 252

thigh and hip fractures, 57–58

third-degree burns, 30

thyroid disease, 136

tibia (lower leg) fractures, 59

toe fractures, 55. *See also* foot, foot problems

tongue, in blocked airway, 157–160

tonsils, 225

toothaches, 257

topical antihistamines, 10

tourniquets, 21, 253

traction, 52, 57

trap squeeze, 66–67

trauma (injury)
    abdominal, 166–170
    altered mental status and, 74

Traveler's diarrhea, 189

trichomonas, 259

triple antibiotic ointment (Neosporin), 10, 109, 256

tubal (ectopic) pregnancy, 196–197

Tylenol (acetaminophen), 256

U

ulcers, 174–175

ulna pulse, 40

umbilical hernia, 184

unconsciousness
    after head trauma, 79
    physical exam, 76–77

upper abdominal quadrants, 172–177

uremia, 73–74

urethritis, 180

urinary tract infections, 180, 258, 259
urine, drinking, 246
uterus, uterus problems
  anatomy, 192–193
  endometriosis, 195
  fibroids, 193
  menstrual cramps, 195–196
  miscarriage, 194
  pelvic inflammatory disease, 194–195
  signs of, 193

V

vaccinations, 4, 154, 224
vagina, vaginal problems
  abnormal bleeding, 200
  cysts, 200
  discharge, 198
  vaginosis, 198–199
  yeast infections, 199–200, 256
vagus nerve, 83
Valsalva maneuver, 136–137
Vaseline petroleum jelly, 30, 251, 257
vasovagal syncope, 83
ventricular fibrillation (V-fib), 128
vertigo, 118–122
vitamin D, 9, 196
vitamin deficiencies, 257
vitamins B_1, B_6, 196
vomiting
  of blood, 175
  dehydration from, 188

W

warts, 14–15
wasp stings, 100–101
water
  alternate fluids, 246
  disinfecting, 240–243
  emergency purification supplies,
    254–255
  emergency supplies of, 6, 240
  removing chemicals from, 244–245
  solar still, 243

water filters, 242–243
weather hazards. *See* elements (weather)
whooping cough, 258
witch hazel, 34
Wolff-Parkinson-White syndrome, 136
women's health
  anatomy, 192–193
  bimanual exam (pelvic exam), 194
  emergency childbirth, 201–206
  fallopian tubes, 196–197
  ovaries, 197–198
  quiz, 191–192
  uterus, 192–196
  vagina, 198–200
wounds
  bleeding control, 19–21
  cleaning, 22–23
  closing, 21–22, 23–25
  eye wounds, 108
  honey for, 26, 257
  puncture wounds, 26–27, 166–168
  scalp wounds, 25
  sucking chest wound, 151–152
  sugar for, 26
  unsticking bandage from, 252
  when to get help, 23
wrist fractures, 1–2, 54–55

Y

yeast infection (vaginal), 199–200, 256
yogurt, for yeast infections, 199

Z

Zantac (ranitidine), 256
Zithromax (azithromycin), 99, 258
Zoloft, 139
Z-Pak (azithromycin), 99, 258

ACKNOWLEDGMENTS

Thank you, Andrea Au Levitt, for your patience and guidance, and for giving me the opportunity to write for Reader's Digest. And to Barbara Clark, thanks for your editing skills, which have made the book so much better than it would have been otherwise.

Thanks to Joe M. Ruiz for the great illustrations, which add artful clarity.

Thanks to my agent, Linda Konner, who has had faith in my writing and worked diligently to find the publisher that fit me the best.

Thanks to my older daughter, Leigh Ann, an editor who from the beginning has helped me put my doctor-speak into plain English so everyone can better understand what I'm trying to say.

Thanks to my wife, Pam, and to my younger daughter, Beth, for sharing their knowledge in areas where I most need help.

Thanks to my colleagues, including physicians and other health care professionals, and to my patients who have taught me so much through the years.

ABOUT THE AUTHOR

James Hubbard never liked hunting. Growing up in Mississippi, he spent many an hour in a deer blind with his dad, but what he really wanted to do was become a doctor.

So he did. But after more than 30 years of practicing family medicine in Mississippi and Colorado, James combined his medical training with his outdoorsy roots to become one of the nation's top survival-medicine experts. He now publishes the number-one survival-medicine website, TheSurvivalDoctor.com, and is the author of *Living Ready Pocket Manual: First Aid,* among other books. His evidence-based tips are a combination of modern medicine, makeshift treatments, and Grandma's home remedies—some of which he witnessed while treating patients from rural areas who couldn't get to a doctor right away.

A graduate of the University of Mississippi School of Medicine, he trained at the acclaimed Parkland Memorial Hospital in Dallas and also earned a master's in public health. A member of the American Academy of Family Physicians, American College of Occupational and Environmental Medicine, American Medical Association, and Wilderness Medical Society, Dr. Hubbard now runs a private practice in Oxford, Mississippi.